The Celiac Disease Diet Plan

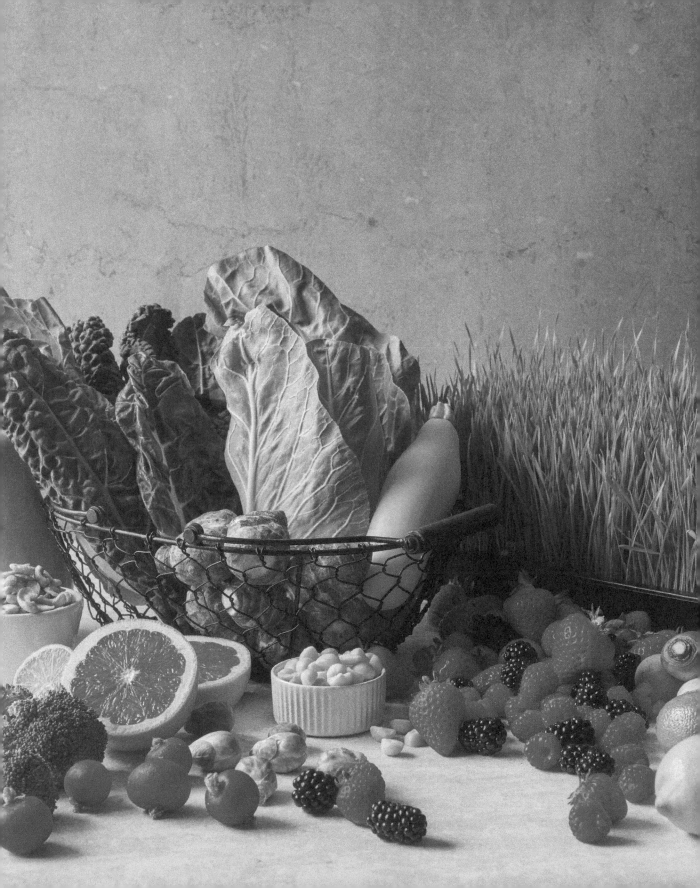

THE
Celiac Disease Diet Plan

YOUR GUIDE TO A HEALTHY GLUTEN-FREE LIFESTYLE

JAMIE FEIT, MS, RD

ROCKRIDGE PRESS

For general information on our other products
and services or to obtain technical support,
please contact our Customer Care Department
within the United States at (866) 744-2665, or
outside the United States at (510) 253-0500.

Rockridge Press publishes its books in a variety
of electronic and print formats. Some content that
appears in print may not be available in electronic
books, and vice versa.

TRADEMARKS: Rockridge Press and the
Rockridge Press logo are trademarks or registered
trademarks of Callisto Media Inc. and/or its
affiliates, in the United States and other countries,
and may not be used without written permission.
All other trademarks are the property of their
respective owners. Rockridge Press is not
associated with any product or vendor mentioned
in this book.

Interior and Cover Designer: Erik Jacobsen
Art Producer: Sara Feinstein
Editor: Sam Eichner
Production Manager: Martin Worthington
Production Editor: Melissa Edeburn
Photography © 2019 Helene Dujardin, cover, p. 14,
26, 42, 52, 62, 80, 96, 110, 126; Darren Muir, p. ii;
2018 Nadine Greeff, p. v-vi, 2; Cayla Zahoran, p.
xii, 40.
Food styling by Anna Hampton, cover, p. ii, xii, 14,
26, 40, 42, 51-52, 62, 80, 96, 110, 126.
Author photo courtesy of © Roger Del Russo.

ISBN: Print 978-1-64611-289-0
Ebook 978-1-64611-290-6
R0

This book is dedicated to my daughter Hannah, who has become a spunky, considerate, thoughtful little girl after many years of random medical symptoms—which turned out to be the result of celiac disease.

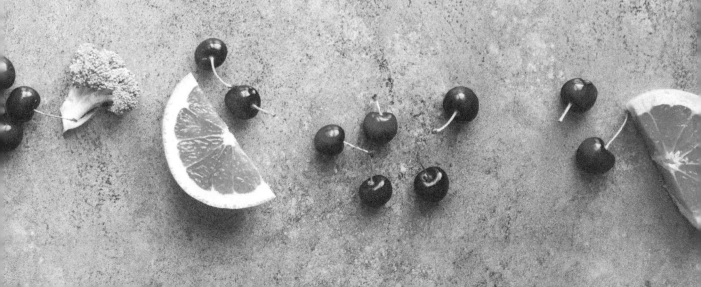

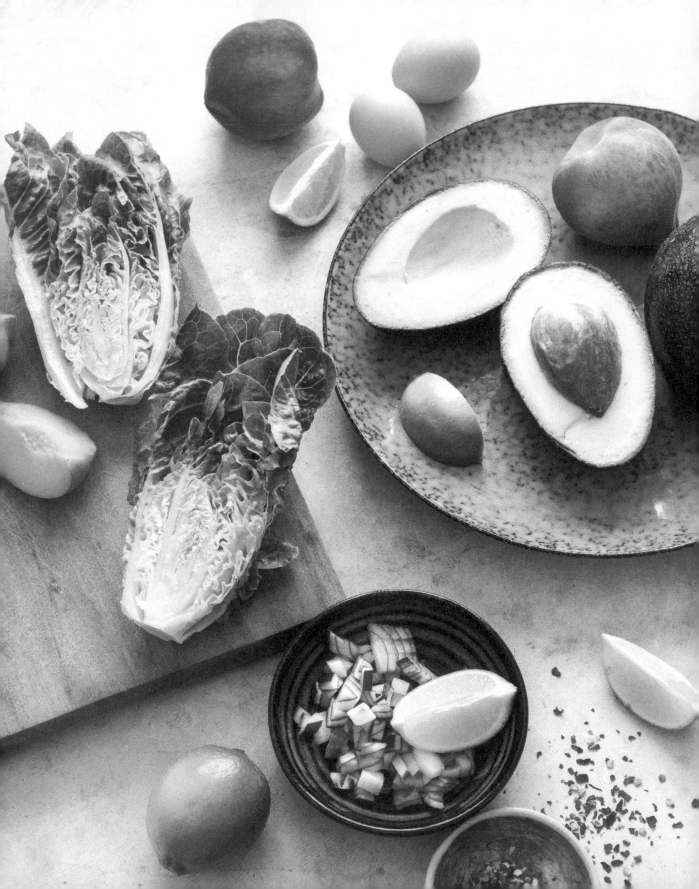

CONTENTS

INTRODUCTION

After three years of seemingly random, unexplained medical symptoms—
like tingling in her hands and feet at night, insomnia, and growth delays—my
seven-year-old daughter Hannah was diagnosed with celiac disease. Thus began our
gluten-free journey—one that was difficult at first, but has since become a natural part
of both my and Hannah's life.

If you or a loved one has recently been diagnosed with celiac disease, I understand
the fear. I understand the trepidation. I understand how overwhelming the changes
may sound and how much more challenging life may seem. I've been a nutritionist for
more than 20 years, and even as a health professional, with a wealth of experience and
knowledge, I, too, experienced these feelings. I'm here to tell you I was there, like so
many others. But I'm also here to help make the transition to gluten-free living as
smooth as possible.

The good news is that a celiac-disease diagnosis has a clear solution—a definitive
end to the painful, uncomfortable symptoms you or your loved one's been experiencing.

There's no medicine to take; all you have to do is completely remove gluten from your diet. This task is, of course, easier said than done. A gluten-free diet is not so much a diet as a lifestyle change.

This book is designed to help lay the groundwork for that lifestyle change. And to be clear: This book is not *just* a gluten-free cookbook. Gluten-free cookbooks are great—I own a few myself—but they don't necessarily provide the information that celiacs, in particular, require—for example, how to scan food labels for evidence of gluten, how to gluten-proof your kitchen, and how to avoid triggering symptoms while traveling and eating at restaurants.

To help kickstart your transition to gluten-free eating, I present, in chapter 3, a two-week meal plan made up of recipes from chapters 4 through 10.

If you stick to the plan, and continue to eat gluten-free, your body will begin to heal. Before you know it, you'll feel better than ever. So, say goodbye to gluten—and say hello to your gluten-free lifestyle!

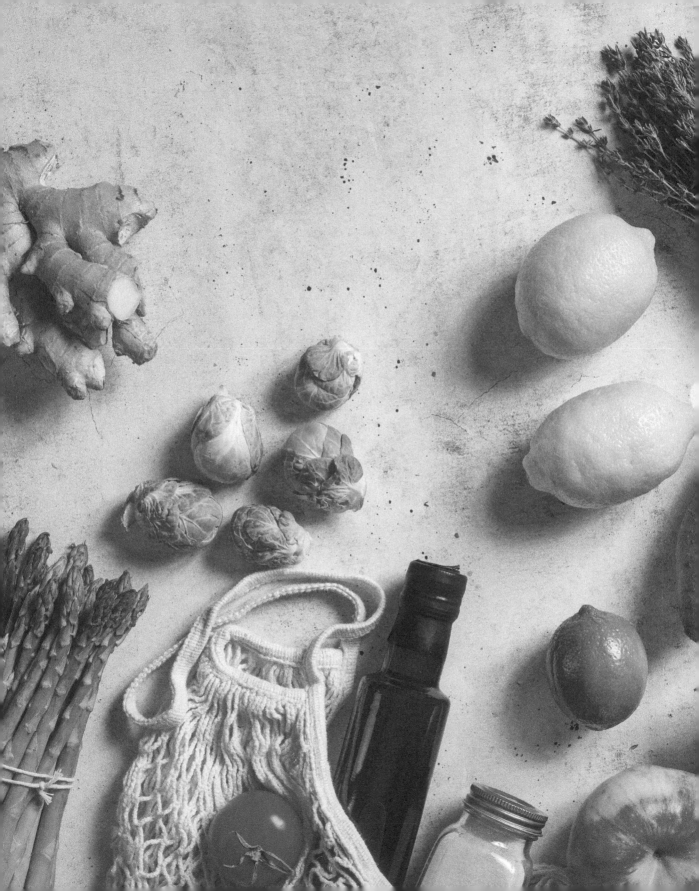

PART ONE

Welcome to the Gluten-Free Lifestyle

In these first few chapters, I'll give you a comprehensive introduction to celiac disease and your new gluten-free lifestyle. In chapter 1, I provide a detailed summary of the disease—what it is, why it's so hard to diagnose, how to make peace with it, and more. In chapter 2, I outline how to completely gluten-proof your home. And in chapter 3, I start you off on an easy-to-follow, two-week gluten-free meal plan, which incorporates the delicious recipes from part 2.

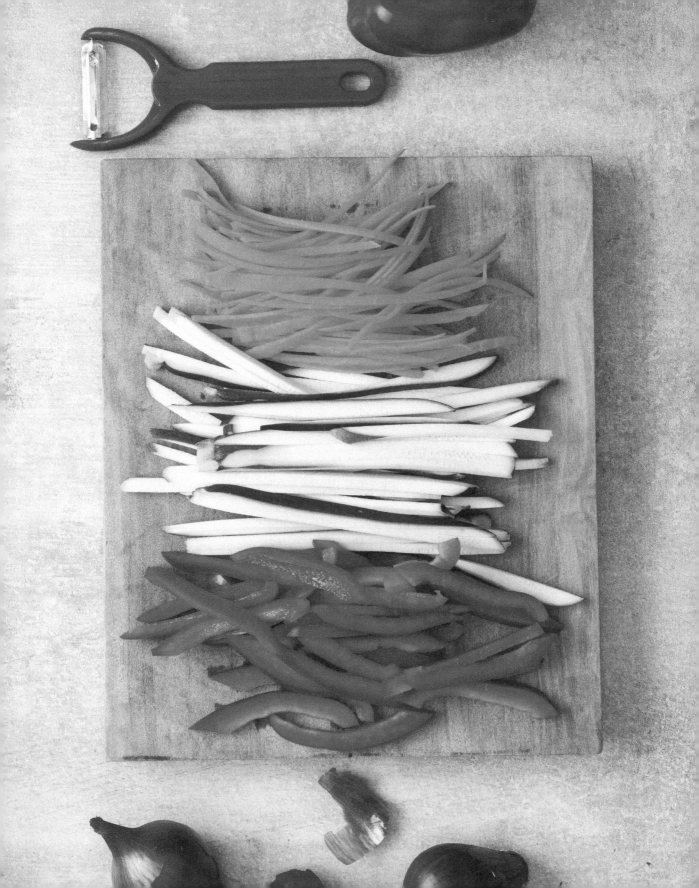

CHAPTER ONE

Demystifying Celiac Disease

One of the scariest aspects of any diagnosis is the unknown. In this chapter, I explain how celiac disease affects the body, why it can be difficult to diagnose, and the conditions that can arise if it goes untreated. In addition, I address common misconceptions about the disease and delve into the science behind those infamous little protein molecules known as gluten.

WHAT WE TALK ABOUT WHEN WE TALK ABOUT CELIAC DISEASE

Celiac disease is an autoimmune disorder. A healthy immune system will destroy potentially harmful substances in your body, preventing you from getting sick. But if you have an autoimmune disorder, your immune system will attack healthy cells by mistake. In the case of celiac disease, the immune system mistakes gluten—protein molecules found in wheat, rye, and barely—for harmful substances. As a result, every time someone with the disease consumes gluten, the immune system ends up attacking the small intestine, where most of the digestion and absorption of food takes place.

In addition to the uncomfortable symptoms this systemic response can cause, such as bloating, gas, diarrhea, and vomiting, these attacks, if ongoing, can damage the small intestine. The small intestine is lined with tiny, hair-like projections called villi, which help the body absorb nutrients as food passes through the digestive system. If a person with celiac disease continues to consume gluten, the villi will become flattened, making digesting and absorbing food harder for the body. The consequences vary, but they may include electrolyte imbalance, vitamin deficiency, significant weight loss, and even depression (see page 7).

Diagnosing celiac disease can be challenging because not everyone shows the same symptoms—or any symptoms at all. For example, some people lose weight with no gastrointestinal effects, whereas others can have terrible gastrointestinal symptoms for years before the cause is identified.

WHAT WE TALK ABOUT WHEN WE TALK ABOUT GLUTEN

Gluten is a protein molecule found not only in wheat, but also in rye, barley, farro, wheat berries, couscous, and some ancient wheats (like einkorn and spelt). Many popular foods made with these grains have gluten, including bread, pizza, bagels, and pasta (see page 16). Gluten helps foods maintain their shape by acting as a glue. It's also what prompts the celiac's immune system to attack itself.

The only way to treat celiac disease is to remove gluten entirely from your diet. The good news is that the human body is resilient. Once gluten is removed from the diet, the body can regenerate and heal the small intestine. Symptoms will improve almost immediately; eventually, they will disappear entirely. As of now, however, there is no cure for celiac disease. (A vaccine trial underway in 2018 has been discontinued.)

You may have heard about people who have chosen to go on a "gluten-free" diet, though they have no gluten-related problems. There are only three reasons to avoid gluten: You have celiac disease, you have a gluten allergy, or you have a gluten sensitivity. Worth noting is the fact that weight loss is *not* on this list. If you're on a diet to lose weight, you may naturally consume less gluten, because gluten is found in many high-calorie, processed foods; similarly, some people who follow a strict, gluten-free diet may consume fewer high-calorie carbs. But a completely gluten-free diet is not, by itself, an effective diet or weight-loss plan. In fact, some of the processed, gluten-free alternatives found in supermarkets have just as many, if not more, calories and fats than the products they're manufactured to replace.

A misperception is that carbohydrates and white-flour products are bad for you. In fact, many carbohydrates are good for you—especially those containing fiber. The "problem" carbohydrates are the ones found in sugary and highly processed foods.

GLUTEN DID THAT

In food, gluten plays five major roles:

- It gives products like bagels their doughy consistency.

- It provides elasticity to bread, muffins, and cakes.

- It creates the air pockets in baked goods, resulting in a light, fluffy texture.

- It enhances flavor.

- It acts as a thickening agent in cooking.

WHO GETS CELIAC DISEASE (AND WHY IT CAN BE SO HARD TO DIAGNOSE)

Celiac disease has been around in one form or another for thousands of years—a Greek physician by the name of Aretaeus of Cappadocia wrote about "The Coeliac Affection" in the first century AD. But it wasn't until the 1960s that the current understanding of the condition emerged. Before then, as an article on the history of the disease from the University of Chicago Celiac Disease Center notes, celiac was considered a rare disease about which doctors knew relatively little.

According to the latest figures from the University of Chicago Celiac Disease Center, the disease affects about 1 percent of healthy, average Americans—meaning at least 3 million people, across all ages, races, and genders, in the United States are living with celiac disease. Some researchers suggest that number may be even higher: A recent study published in *Gastroenterology* estimated the true prevalence was more than 3 percent by age 15. Although the medical community's ability to diagnose the disease has improved, a vast majority of cases remain undiagnosed. Critically, there has been a general uptick in celiac disease, both in the United States and around the world—a phenomenon *The Scientist* dubbed "The Celiac Surge." Though this increase may be attributable to a variety of environmental factors, the underlying causes have not been definitively identified.

Like other autoimmune diseases, celiac has genetic components. If a relative of yours has the disease, your chances of getting it are higher—and you should get tested (see page 8).

Although doctors have become more adept at diagnosing celiac, many still don't consider the disease when evaluating patients' medical complaints. To be fair, the disease can be tricky to diagnose because the symptoms vary so widely among patients. Doctors commonly confuse the symptoms of celiac with those of irritable bowel syndrome. Moreover, patients in our medical system usually go to a physician with one complaint ("I have strep throat") and receive treatment for that single complaint ("Here's an antibiotic"). But celiac disease manifests in many ways, which makes identifying it difficult for doctors.

I know how discouraging looking for a medical answer can be. You know something is very wrong, but your doctors don't seem to take the situation seriously or just can't figure out the cause. Please know that you are not alone. I've been there. This discouragement is one of the reasons I wrote this book. My hope is to provide information that so many people dealing with celiac disease have sorely lacked.

It's All Relative: Celiac Disease and Associated Conditions

When celiac disease goes untreated, other conditions can arise. This list includes some of the most common ones.

Anemia This condition denotes an iron deficiency caused by damage to the intestines. When the intestines are damaged, they cannot absorb iron properly. Because recovery may take a while, you might want to consider taking a supplement for some time after your diagnosis.

Depression Feeling low can be a pervasive side effect of feeling irritable, angry, frustrated, and generally unwell from symptoms of celiac disease.

Osteoporosis A damaged small intestine makes absorbing calcium difficult. For kids, osteoporosis can stunt growth; for an adult, it can reduce bone density. A lack of calcium absorption can cause dental problems as well, potentially leading to dental formation issues.

Dermatitis Herpetiformis
A severe rash can develop in some people with celiac disease. The skin can become incredibly itchy and blister and scab, and the rash does not respond to topical treatments.

Reproductive Problems Left undiagnosed, celiac disease can lead to infertility and complications during pregnancy. The reasons for these issues are not well understood in the medical community, but according to a journal article in *Women's Health*, these problems can be caused by a disruption in the development of reproductive hormones, as well as by nutritional deficiencies.

Migraines These severe headaches are also widespread among people with undiagnosed celiac disease. They can be triggered by abnormalities in blood flow to the brain, due to lack of nutrient absorption.

HOW TO TELL IF YOU HAVE CELIAC DISEASE

The only way to know for certain that you have celiac disease is to receive a diagnosis from your doctor. To make that diagnosis, your doctor will need to perform three tests. The first is a blood test to determine whether your immune system is mistakenly sending out antibodies to attack the gluten in your body. The second is an endoscopy, a nonsurgical procedure used to examine the digestive tract. The third is a biopsy of the small intestine, which is used to evaluate the condition of the villi.

If you have celiac disease, your blood test will be positive for antibodies and your endoscopy, biopsy, or both will show damage to the small intestine.

It's not uncommon to receive mixed results from these tests. For example, your blood test could come back positive for the antibodies fighting off gluten, whereas your biopsy could come back negative, showing no damage to the intestine. In this case, you would not be diagnosed with celiac disease, but your doctor might diagnose you with a gluten sensitivity, which could lead to celiac disease.

If you're tempted to forgo a trip to the doctor, beware the dangers of self-diagnosis and treatment. If, say, you've decided you are gluten sensitive, but you are not sticking to a 100 percent gluten-free diet, you could be setting yourself up to develop lifelong medical problems from undiagnosed celiac disease. Make an appointment with your doctor right away, and use the list of symptoms in the following section to help explain why you would like a blood test for the disease.

SIGNS YOU MAY HAVE CELIAC DISEASE

If you frequently experience more than one of the following symptoms, for no discernible reason, you could have celiac disease and you may want to get tested. I've listed the most common symptoms—some of which you may not typically associate with celiac disease.

- Anemia
- Bloating
- Bone/dental malformation
- Depression
- Diarrhea

- Gas
- Headache
- Joint pain
- Mouth sores
- Nausea, vomiting, or both

- Skin rash
- Stomach cramps
- Tingling of the extremities
- Unexplained weight loss
- Vitamin deficiencies

Take Your Vitamins

Undiagnosed, celiac disease could lead to a deficiency in essential vitamins and minerals, due to the small intestine's inability to properly absorb nutrients. In particular, some B vitamins like folic acid (critical for reproduction and during pregnancy), fat-soluble vitamins (key for calcium absorption and blood clotting), and iron (necessary for the production of red blood cells) may be severely depleted. The intestine will start to repair itself as soon as gluten is removed from the diet, but a return to function can take time.

So, if you have been diagnosed with the disease, you should absolutely get a blood test to see whether you have any severe vitamin deficiencies. If you do, supplements may be warranted, though you should discuss these with your doctor or a registered dietician. In any event, you'll want to include varied servings of four fruits and four vegetables in your daily diet to provide the vitamins the body needs as it heals.

I recommend taking a daily multivitamin immediately after being diagnosed (naturally, you'll want to choose one that does not contain gluten!). As the villi in the small intestine are regenerated, the intestines will start absorbing nutrients at a normal level, at which point you may no longer find the vitamin necessary.

MAKING PEACE WITH YOUR DIAGNOSIS

It can be difficult to come to terms with a diagnosis for a disease with no cure—especially one that can have such a significant effect on your everyday life. To feel shock, anger, disbelief, worry, and frustration is absolutely natural. But a diagnosis can also come as a relief after what may have been years of pain and discomfort. Finally, you have a definitive problem—and, most importantly, a proven solution.

I do not have celiac disease. My daughter, however, was diagnosed at seven years old, even though she had never experienced any gastrointestinal symptoms. She had always been small, but was growing steadily. Yet, strangely enough, she had such severe tingling in her hands and feet that she would wake up in the middle of the night. I took her to no less than 10 physicians, none of whom could tell us what was wrong. Each one had a different diagnosis. Ultimately, she was prescribed sleeping pills to get her to sleep through the night.

Needless to say, this situation was incredibly frustrating. There is nothing worse than knowing something is very wrong with your child, only to find that medical professionals are not taking your concern seriously. People with celiac disease, and other unexplained medical issues, know this experience all too often. As a health professional, I'm very knowledgeable about the gastrointestinal side effects and dietary treatment for celiac disease. Even so, I never connected the dots with the symptoms my daughter showed.

Fortunately, one doctor—who happened to be my eldest daughter's endocrinologist—picked up on the tingling in my daughter's extremities. She walked me across the hall, introduced me to a gastroenterologist, and told me she was positive she had celiac disease. Sure enough, the endoscopy revealed that the villi on her intestines were completely flat. Now, after two-and-a-half years without gluten, she is completely healthy.

At first, your own diagnosis—or the diagnosis of a loved one—may come as a shock. But I would implore you to focus less on the frustration and anger and more on the relief and comfort that comes with knowing that there is, finally, an explanation for your symptoms. With a little time and dedication, a gluten-free diet plan—like the one I detail in chapter 3—will help you start to feel better. You may even feel like you have a brand new lease on life!

THE BENEFITS OF A GLUTEN-FREE DIET

Being diagnosed with celiac disease requires going gluten-free and giving up many foods, such as pizza, pasta, cakes, doughnuts, pastries, and bagels. Eating in restaurants becomes problematic, as does picking up packaged foods at convenience stores (see page 16). But if there's a silver lining to having celiac disease, it's that a gluten-free diet is generally a healthy diet—provided you avoid processed gluten-free products that can be high in both calories and fat. If you approach this lifestyle change as an opportunity to consume more gluten-free whole grains, fruits, vegetables, and lean protein, your overall diet will improve.

In the next chapter, I'll help you fill your gluten-free kitchen with healthy whole grains and everything else you'll need to embark on the diet plan laid out in chapter 3.

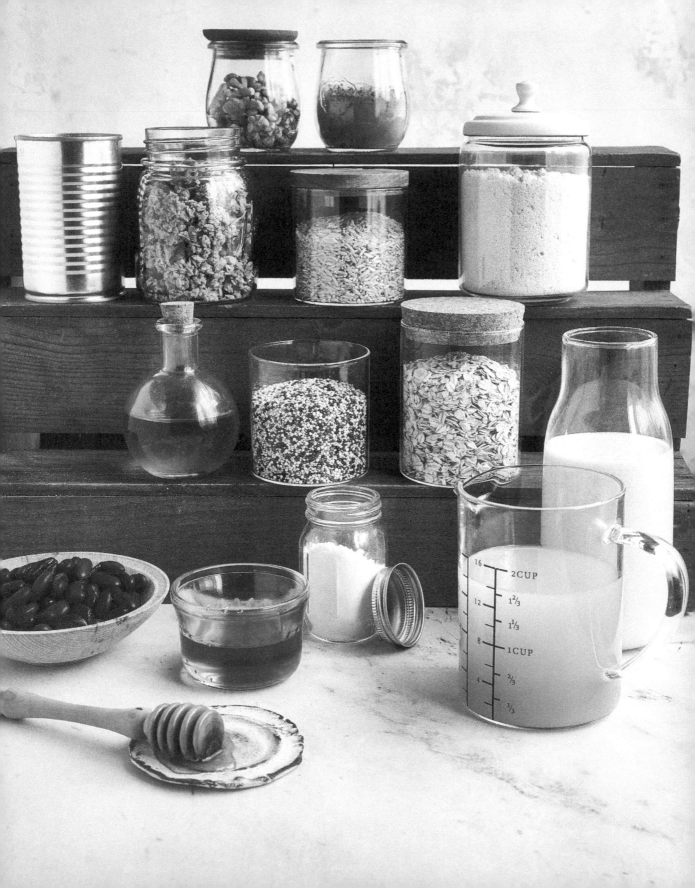

CHAPTER TWO

Gluten-Proofing Your Home

In this chapter, I'll review which foods and ingredients are safe to consume, and which items need to be removed from your kitchen and cooking spaces. I'll also go over how to scan labels for gluten—an invaluable skill that's critical for effectively navigating the supermarket. Building a gluten-free kitchen is totally doable. And once you have a gluten-free kitchen, you'll be ready to prepare all of the delicious, celiac-friendly recipes in part 2 of this book.

WHERE GLUTEN IS HIDING

Gluten is sneaky: It can linger in places you least expect. In the following lists, I'll cover the most common food items and ingredients that contain gluten, as well as those that *might* contain gluten. I'll also cover popular non-food items, like cosmetics, which contain gluten. With some practice and a bit of diligence, identifying items containing gluten will become second nature. (For a more comprehensive list of safe and unsafe ingredients, please refer to the Master List of Safe/Unsafe Ingredients on page 137.)

FOOD ITEMS AND INGREDIENTS WITH GLUTEN

Make sure to avoid all of these items. (If a gluten-free version is available, it must be explicitly marked gluten-free.)

- Barley
- Beer
- Bread
- Bread crumbs
- Bulgur
- Cakes
- Cookies
- Couscous
- Croutons
- Gummy candy
- Licorice
- Pasta
- Pastries
- Pizza
- Pretzels
- Rye
- Seitan (commonly used in vegetarian meals)
- Soy sauce
- Wheat berries
- Wheat bran

FOOD ITEMS AND INGREDIENTS THAT *MIGHT* HAVE GLUTEN

Before eating any of the items on the following list, check the label to make sure they don't contain ingredients with gluten. If you're eating in a restaurant, consult with a waitstaff or chef (see page 37). Most sauces, marinades, and rubs potentially contain gluten, especially if one of the ingredients is soy sauce. Salad dressings can also be problematic. Even packaged products that you would assume are gluten-free, like potato chips, can contain a flavoring or other ingredients with gluten.

- Barbecue sauce
- Blue cheese
- Bouillon
- Imitation bacon bits
- Fried food (due to cross-contamination in the fryer)
- Mashed potato mixes
- Oats
- Packaged snacks (such as potato chips)
- Pickles
- Salad dressings
- Sushi (imitation crab, soy sauce, surimi, tempura flakes, and vinegar can contain wheat)
- Tea
- Teriyaki sauce
- Tomato or marinara sauce
- Seasonings
- Semolina

NON-FOOD ITEMS WITH GLUTEN

It might surprise you to learn that many non-food products contain gluten. If you're taking any vitamins, supplements, or medications, check the label to see if wheat, malt, modified food starch, or caramel color is anywhere on the ingredient list. (Caramel color in the United States is gluten-free, but if a product comes from another country, it might not be.) The inactive ingredients in medications and supplements may contain gluten as well, because starch can be used as a binder.

I realize the list below does not include many specifics. The reason is simply because whether an item contains gluten is subject to change. Therefore, you must be vigilant when checking the labels on these kinds of products.

- Lip glosses
- Lipsticks
- Over-the-counter medications
- Playdough (young children may put it in their mouths or they may put their hands in their mouth after playing with the dough)
- Prescription medications
- Supplements
- Toothpaste
- Vitamins

CHECKING THE LABEL

If you've never read food labels before for nutritional information, you'll need to start once you've been diagnosed with celiac disease. The first place you'll want to look is the allergen section. Since 2013, federal law has mandated that wheat be included in this part of the label, along with other allergens. If you see "wheat," you'll know you must avoid the product. But just because a product does not contain wheat, does not mean the product is gluten-free. Laws do not require other gluten-containing ingredients—such as barley, rye, and spelt—to be listed, so you will still need to become familiar with which ingredients are and are not safe. You should make a habit of reading food labels, even for products you've purchased before. Ingredients can change over time, often without warning.

If the gluten-free product is manufactured on equipment that also processes products that contain gluten, there's a chance that this otherwise gluten-free product has been cross-contaminated. Fortunately, food labels include warnings such as "This product is manufactured in a facility that processes other products which may contain wheat." Additionally, the label will list the ingredients for the other products made in the same processing plant. For example, even though chocolate is gluten-free, a chocolate bar may have a label noting that it might have been processed on the same equipment as a product containing wheat. Some celiacs can tolerate food processed on shared equipment; some cannot. Unfortunately, there is no standardized amount of gluten a celiac can tolerate without producing adverse effects. If a label has this warning, I recommend avoiding the food entirely, unless you know your tolerance level for such foods.

Most supermarkets will have a full list of gluten-free products in their store. I recommend requesting the list from a manager before you begin shopping. Alternatively, you can bring this book along with you, and refer to the Master List of Safe/Unsafe Ingredients on page 137.

GLUTEN ALIASES

Here are some of the most common food labeling terms that suggest the presence of gluten. If you see one of these, make sure you read the label carefully.

- Artificial and natural flavor (may contain barley)

- Brewer's yeast (found in beer)

- Caramel color (typically in products outside the United States)

- Food coloring

- Food flavors

- Fish sauce

- Hydrolyzed wheat protein

- Malt

- Malt vinegar

- Modified food starch (may come from wheat, corn, or soy; only gluten-free if made from corn)

- Vegetable starch (may come from wheat, corn, or soy; only gluten-free if made from corn)

THE GLUTEN-FREE KITCHEN

Setting up your gluten-free kitchen can seem like a daunting task, but it really just takes a little organization and forethought.

First, you'll need to decide whether the entire kitchen will be gluten-free or whether only part of the kitchen will be reserved for gluten-free cooking. Both ways can work; make a choice and stick with it. If you're living on your own, how you arrange your kitchen won't be an issue. But if you're living with a partner, family, or roommates, you'll have to decide how you will approach gluten in your kitchen together. If one or more members of your household want to cook food with gluten, you'll have to be vigilant.

The main problem with a "split" kitchen is the potential for cross-contamination. Contamination can occur when equipment or cookware used to prepare something containing gluten is improperly cleaned. Even trace amounts of gluten can trigger discomfort for some people with celiac disease.

The two items I recommend purchasing for your gluten-free kitchen are mesh strainers and toasters; both tend to trap ingredients containing gluten, and thoroughly cleaning them may be difficult. All other kitchen utensils, pots, pans, cutting boards, knives, and baking dishes can be washed well with soap and water to eradicate any trace of gluten.

Once you've thoroughly cleaned everything, including any surface where you prepare food, you're ready to set up your new kitchen. If you're working with a split kitchen, decide which items will be used for gluten and which will not, then separate them accordingly. If you have the budget, you may want to purchase duplicates of some items, such as a bread knife (although, if washed well, the knife shouldn't pose a problem). You'll also have to determine which areas will be for gluten-containing food. All family members should be clear on how the kitchen will be set up. Naturally, for this setup to work, gluten must be limited to the parts of the kitchen designated for gluten.

You need to make clear to your household that using a utensil for food containing gluten, and then using that same utensil for food that's gluten-free, will result in cross-contamination. For this reason, you may choose to stock duplicates of items like butter, cream cheese, jams, and mustard.

In any event, communication is key. Establishing clear ground rules at the outset will save a lot of time (and hassle) down the road.

In my home, I've found that the best arrangement is about a 90/10 split kitchen—meaning that everything I cook is gluten-free, all my pots, pans, and cooking utensils are gluten-free, and 90 percent of all food in the refrigerator, freezer, and pantry, are gluten-free. The remaining 10 percent of our food consists of clearly labeled butter and cream cheese in the refrigerator, as well as one drawer of food containing gluten in the freezer and one counter we've designated as not gluten-free.

Help, I Love Bread! Or, Which Gluten-Free Substitutes Are Right for Me?

Bread: It's a dreaded word in a celiac's vocabulary. And yes, you may feel like life without it will never be the same. However, there are some excellent substitutes to satisfy these cravings. Keep in mind, as I've mentioned already, that gluten-free food is not necessarily healthy food. Gluten-free products can be heavily processed and high in calories, fat, and gluten-free carbohydrates.

As a nutritionist, I recommend the following gluten-free products—and a few of my own recipes from part 2. You can find these brands in most supermarkets; in the Resources section (see page 142), I've listed websites where these products can be purchased.

Gluten-free beer: Dogfish Head Tweason' Ale, Steadfast Golden Blonde, and Green's Amber Ale

Gluten-free bread: Schär and Canyon Bakehouse products, or my homemade Essential Sandwich Rolls (page 46)

Gluten-free brownie mix: King Arthur Flour Gluten Free Fudge Brownie Mix or my Super Gooey Chocolate Brownies (page 135)

Gluten-free cereal: Cheerios, Chex, Bob's Red Mill oatmeal, and KIND granola

Gluten-free chips: Food Should Taste Good, Kettle Brand, and Slete kettle-cooked potato chips; Beanfields tortilla chips; and Garden of Eatin' products

Gluten-free cookies: Simple Mills, Goodie Girl Cookies, Enjoy Life Foods, and Lucy's products

Gluten-free crackers: Simple Mills, Mary's Gone Crackers, and Schär

Gluten-free muffin mix: Simple Mills

Gluten-free pasta: Barilla, Bionaturae, Tinkyada, and Le Veneziane

Gluten-free pizza dough: Udi's, Caulipower, Mama Mary's, Kinnkinick, and my own Essential Pizza Crust (page 50)

THE GLUTEN-FREE PANTRY

Setting up your gluten-free pantry will ensure you have safe-to-eat food on hand. First, you'll want to remove everything from the pantry and wipe out each shelf to eliminate any gluten. Then, toss out any open items and items that contain gluten, such as certain cereals, breads, crackers, pasta, barley, cookies, snack foods, and sauces. Unopened packages of safe foods may be put back in the pantry after the shelves have been cleaned. I recommend stocking up on the items listed below. Some may be unfamiliar to you, because they're gluten-free substitutes for cooking and baking. But I assure you, these items are both affordable and available at most supermarkets.

- Baking powder
- Baking soda
- Beans, canned
- Broth (chicken, vegetable, or both)
- Cocoa powder
- Coconut milk
- Confectioners' sugar
- Cooking oil spray
- Cornstarch

- Flours (almond, brown rice, and sweet rice, for baking)
- Gluten-free crackers
- Gluten-free granola
- Gluten-free oats
- Gluten-free pasta
- Gluten-free soy sauce
- Honey
- Nuts (almonds, pecans, pistachios, and walnuts)

- Oil (avocado, canola, and olive)
- Quinoa
- Rice
- Salsa
- Sugar
- Tomatoes, canned
- Tomato sauce
- Vanilla extract
- Xanthan gum (for baking)

THE GLUTEN-FREE REFRIGERATOR

To set up your gluten-free refrigerator, be very careful to remove everything from the shelves and wipe them down. Then, toss out any open items that could be contaminated, like butter, jam, or hummus. Take a look at the labels of salad dressings, sauces, yogurts, and the like, and toss out anything that has wheat or gluten-containing ingredients. After the refrigerator is cleaned out, I recommend stocking up on the items listed below.

- Almond butter
- Almond milk
- Butter
- Cheese
- Corn tortillas
- Cream cheese
- Eggs
- Fruit, seasonal
- Garlic
- Gluten-free pickles
- Jam
- Lemons
- Limes
- Milk
- Onions
- Peanut butter
- Vegetables, seasonal
- Yogurt

THE GLUTEN-FREE FREEZER

Almost everyone stores leftovers in the freezer, whether pizza, half-eaten tubs of ice cream, or leftover dinners. A gluten-free freezer should be thoroughly cleaned out. Unless there are unopened products that are definitely gluten-free, you'll want to throw everything out, particularly leftovers, as you likely won't be able to tell if they've come in contact with gluten. After the freezer is cleaned out, I recommend stocking up on the items listed below, which include some of the healthiest, easiest-to-use frozen fruits and veggies.

- Frozen berries
- Frozen cauliflower
- Frozen edamame
- Frozen meat and fish
- Frozen spinach
- Gluten-free frozen bread or rolls (see Essential Sandwich Rolls, page 46)
- Gluten-free ice cream

THE KITCHEN EQUIPMENT

Now that you (or a loved one) must remain gluten-free, the safest place to eat is at home. Acquiring the right equipment will make gluten-free cooking that much easier. I've created two lists: One list contains the tools necessary to make the recipes in this book; the other contains tools that, although not absolutely necessary, will help you prepare the recipes more efficiently.

Must Have

- Baking dishes, glass (8-by-8-inch and 9-by-13-inch)
- Blender
- Cutting boards
- Hand mixer
- Knives, full set
- Mason jars
- Measuring cups and spoons
- Mixing bowls
- Mixing spoons
- Muffin tins
- Parchment paper (for baking)
- Pots and saucepans, full set
- Resealable bags or containers
- Rolling pin
- Sheet pans
- Skillets (ideally 8-, 10-, and 12-inch)
- Spatulas
- Whisk

Nice to Have

- Food processor
- Garlic press
- Immersion blender
- Indoor grill pan or outdoor grill
- Loaf pans (for making gluten-free bread)
- Pizza stone (for making pizza crust)
- Potato masher
- Spiralizer
- Stand mixer (for making dough)
- Toaster
- Waffle pan or iron
- Wire racks (for cooling baked goods)
- Zester

Celiac Disease and Lactose Intolerance

Lactose intolerance is a condition in which a person lacks the enzyme necessary to break down lactose, which is the carbohydrate found in dairy products. If lactose is not digested by the time it moves along the digestive tract to the small intestine, it can cause gas, stomach cramps, and bloating until it is absorbed by the villi of the small intestine.

In some celiac patients with damaged villi, lactose cannot be digested. Although the cause of the resulting lactose intolerance is not a missing enzyme, the condition can still be treated by taking lactase pills or by avoiding dairy products. Many of the recipes in this book are dairy-free, and are clearly labeled as such; many others offer dairy-free substitutes. Essential to point out: Once gluten is removed from the diet and the intestine is repaired, the lactose intolerance may disappear—if, in fact, this intolerance was caused by celiac and not the missing enzyme.

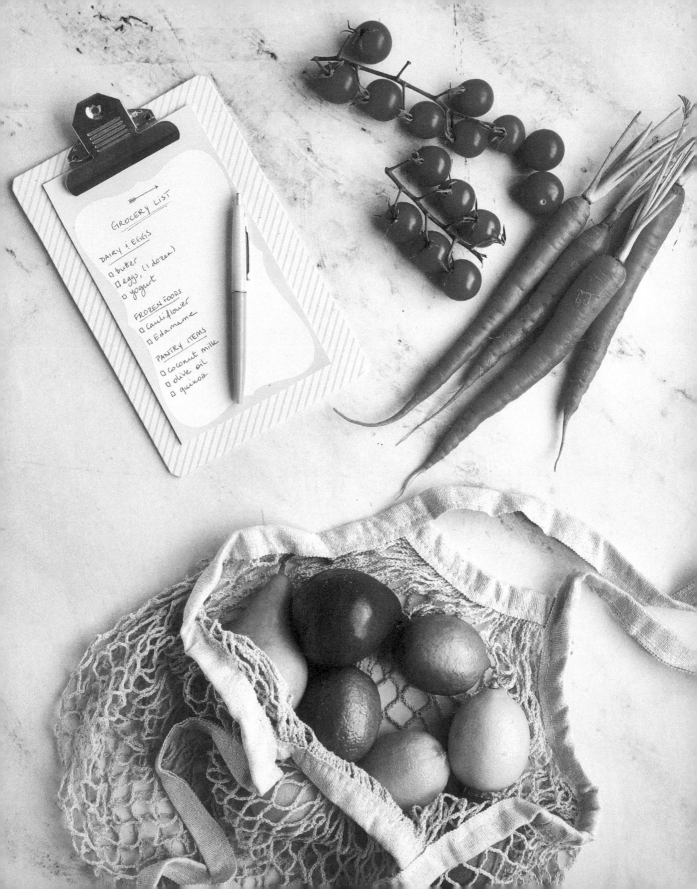

GROCERY LIST

DAIRY & EGGS

□ butter
□ eggs (1 dozen)
□ yogurt

FROZEN FOODS

□ cauliflower
□ Edamame

PANTRY ITEMS

□ coconut milk
□ olive oil
□ quinoa

CHAPTER THREE

The Happy, Healthy, Gluten-Free Meal Plan

When you have celiac disease, going gluten-free is not simply a diet—it's a lifestyle. Although this change may seem daunting, it's much easier to accomplish once you know how to get started. That's why I've created this comprehensive, easy-to-use, 14-day meal plan, complete with simple snacks, meal prep tips, and delicious recipes from throughout the book. In addition, I've provided some strategies for eating gluten-free outside of your own home. Think of this chapter as a springboard, launching you safely into a healthy gluten-free life.

WEEK ONE

This meal plan is designed to make eating tasty, nutritious gluten-free food as easy and stress-free as possible. Although following the plan for the first week is likely to be the most challenging, you'll learn how to prepare delicious gluten-free food, and you'll discover how simple and enjoyable gluten-free living can be!

Week One Meal Plan Prep

Following my weekly meal plan is easy—and it will be even easier if you put in a bit of prep work. Here are some tips to make sure everything goes according to plan during your first week:

1. **This meal plan is designed for two people.**
   If you're using this meal plan for yourself or for four people, you can make adjustments accordingly; to halve or double recipes, simply cut the ingredients in half or double them, and follow the recipes as written.

   This is your meal plan: If you think you'll want more than one serving, make more; if you think you'll want less, make less.

2. **Note the leftover suggestions.**
   Several recipes show up in the meal plan twice (and a few from Week One show up in Week Two). The first time, it's recommended two servings are consumed; the second time, you'll notice a "leftover" notation, and it's recommended the other two servings are consumed. For example, Caramelized Onion and Mushroom Pizza

is listed for dinner on Wednesday night, and Leftover Caramelized Onion and Mushroom Pizza is listed for lunch on Friday. In this instance, it's recommended that half the pizza be eaten on Wednesday night and that the rest be shared on Friday. Leftovers can be stored in airtight containers or resealable bags in the refrigerator.

If there are leftovers from meals or sides that aren't listed in the meal plan, they can be stored in the refrigerator and finished whenever you like; alternatively, most recipes will remain good for a few months if frozen in a freezer-friendly container.

3. **Make sure you have all the kitchen equipment needed to prepare the recipes.**
   The essentials are listed in chapter 2 (see page 24), but having the following equipment on hand will make preparing this week's recipes especially painless:

   - Baking dishes, glass (8-by-8- and 9-by-13-inch)

- Blender
- Hand mixer
- Mason jars
- Mixing bowls
- Muffin tins
- Saucepans
- Sheet pans
- Skillets (medium and large)

4. **Do your grocery shopping on Sunday.**
Go through the menus on the meal plan, create a grocery list, and then head out to the grocery store. Be sure to include:

- All non-perishable items. You can store them in your pantry.

- Ingredients for the Mediterranean Egg Cups (page 56), the week's desserts, and any perishable ingredients you'll require for the first four days. You can either return to the store mid-week for the rest of the perishable ingredients, or buy them on Sunday and freeze the meat and fish you don't use the first four days.

- Fruits and vegetables for snacks, plus Greek yogurt for a quick, no-hassle breakfast.

- Enough gluten-free snacks for two weeks (see meal plan for recommendations).

5. **Prepare a few items after you're done shopping on Sunday.**
Getting these tasks out of the way will save you a significant amount of time during the week:

- Cut up veggies (for snacks) and store in resealable bags or airtight containers in the refrigerator.

- Prepare one batch of Mediterranean Egg Cups and refrigerate them for quick breakfasts on Monday, Wednesday, and Friday.

- Bake one or more desserts ahead of time, if you foresee not having as much time during the week: Super Gooey Chocolate Brownies (page 135), Peanut Butter Chocolate Chip Cookies (page 131), and Dark Chocolate Bark with Pumpkin and Pecans (page 134). These can be enjoyed during Week Two (and beyond, if frozen) as well!

- Prepare the Essential Pizza Crust dough and bake the Essential Sandwich Rolls (page 46); you'll need them for the week ahead, and the rolls you can serve with soups, the Zesty Scallion Turkey Burgers (page 112), and leftovers.

6. **Consider the recipes you'll need to prep the day before you'll eat them.**
Make Peanut Butter and Jelly Overnight Oats (page 58) on Monday and Friday to be ready Tuesday and Saturday morning. To serve two, you'll need to double this recipe.

And, of course, if there are lunch recipes you won't have time to make the day-of, do your best to make them ahead of time!

WEEK ONE MEAL PLAN

DAY #	BREAKFAST	LUNCH	DINNER	SNACKS AND DESSERT
Day 1 Monday	4 Mediterranean Egg Cups	Sweet Red Pepper Gazpacho Spicy Cucumber Salad	Shirataki Noodles with Turkey Sausage Arugula Salad with Pomegranate Seeds and Pears	**Snacks:** Carrot sticks and hummus Gluten-free pretzels **Dessert:** Super Gooey Chocolate Brownies Fruit
Day 2 Tuesday	Peanut Butter and Jelly Overnight Oats	Portobello Mushroom Pizza	Quinoa Stuffed Peppers Leftover Spicy Cucumber Salad	**Snacks:** Celery sticks with peanut butter or almond butter Popcorn **Dessert:** Peanut Butter Chocolate Chip Cookies Fruit
Day 3 Wednesday	4 Mediterranean Egg Cups	Leftover Shirataki Noodles with Turkey Sausage	Caramelized Onion and Mushroom Pizza Leftover Sweet Red Pepper Gazpacho	**Snacks:** Cherry tomatoes Veggie straws **Dessert:** Dark Chocolate Bark with Pumpkin and Pecans Fruit
Day 4 Thursday	Greek yogurt with fruit and nuts	Leftover Quinoa Stuffed Peppers	Red Curry Salmon Aromatic Vegetable Quinoa	**Snacks:** Sliced cucumbers with hummus 2 gluten-free granola bars **Dessert:** Peanut Butter Chocolate Chip Cookies Fruit

DAY #	BREAKFAST	LUNCH	DINNER	SNACKS AND DESSERT
Day 5 Friday	4 Mediterranean Egg Cups	Leftover Caramelized Onion and Mushroom Pizza	Roasted Olive Chicken Healthy Cauliflower Fried Rice	**Snacks:** Mini peppers Potato chips **Dessert:** Super Gooey Chocolate Brownies Fruit
Day 6 Saturday	Peanut Butter and Jelly Overnight Oats	Hawaiian Tofu Kabobs	Rosemary-Crusted Lamb Carrot and Ginger Spiced Rice	**Snacks:** Celery sticks with peanut butter or almond butter Tortilla chips **Dessert:** Dark Chocolate Bark with Pumpkin and Pecans Fruit
Day 7 Sunday	Banana Pancakes	Leftover Roasted Olive Chicken	Zesty Scallion Turkey Burgers Spiced Peas	**Snacks:** Apple slices 2 gluten-free granola bars **Dessert:** Super Gooey Chocolate Brownie Fruit

WEEK TWO

Congrats! You've successfully gone through your first week. I'm sure sticking to the meal plan was challenging, but I can assure you doing so only gets easier. Last week, you got used to preparing gluten-free food and planning your meals. This week, you'll solidify what you've learned. By the end, I hope you'll have found some meals you're willing to repeat in the future. More importantly, I hope you'll have grown more confident in preparing gluten-free food at home.

Week Two Meal Plan Prep

Here are some tips to make sure everything goes according to plan during your second week:

1. **Take note of the recipes from Week One used during Week Two.**
   This week's recipes include leftover Hawaiian Tofu Kabobs, Carrot and Ginger Spiced Rice, and Dark Chocolate Bark with Pumpkin and Pecans—plus any unlisted leftovers you may've accumulated!

2. **Make sure you have all the kitchen equipment needed to prepare the recipes.**
   The essentials are listed in chapter 2 (see page 24), but having the following equipment on hand will make preparing this week's recipes especially painless:

   - Baking dish, glass (9-by-13-inch)
   - Blender
   - Hand mixer
   - Mixing bowls
   - Saucepans
   - Sheet pans
   - Skillets (medium and large)
   - Stockpot
   - Waffle pan or iron

3. **Do your grocery shopping on Sunday.**
   Just as you did for Week One, plan to look over the menu, create a shopping list, and head to the grocery store on Sunday. With your provisions in hand, you'll be able to prepare some meals and snacks ahead of time. Make sure to purchase the following:

   - All non-perishable items. You can store them in your pantry.
   - Ingredients for the Chocolate-Banana Baked Oatmeal (page 61), the week's desserts, and any perishable ingredients you'll require for the first four days. You can either return to the store mid-week for the rest of the perishable ingredients, or buy them on Sunday

and freeze the meat and fish you don't use the first four days.

- Fruits and vegetables for snacks, plus Greek yogurt for a quick, no-hassle breakfast.

- More gluten-free snacks (as needed).

4. **Prepare a few items after you're done shopping on Sunday.**
Getting these tasks out of the way will save you a significant amount of time during the week:

- Cut up veggies (for snacks) and store in resealable bags or airtight containers in the refrigerator.

- Prepare the Chocolate-Banana Baked Oatmeal recipe and refrigerate the squares for breakfast Monday, Wednesday, and Friday.

- Bake the Meringue Cookies (page 130) and/or Dark Chocolate Bark with Pumpkin and Pecans (page 134) ahead of time, if you

foresee not having as much time during the week.

- Bake any additional Essential Sandwich Rolls (page 46), which you can serve with soups, the Mexican Salmon Burgers (page 99), and leftovers.

5. **Consider the recipes you need to start the day or night previous.**
If you're making Chocolate Mousse (page 133) for dessert (on Friday and Sunday), refrigerate the can of coconut milk the night before so the cream and liquid separate. Chill the Overnight Marinated Broccoli (page 75) on Saturday so that it's ready for Sunday.

If there are lunch recipes you won't have time to make the day-of, do your best to make them ahead of time!

WEEK TWO MEAL PLAN

DAY #	BREAKFAST	LUNCH	DINNER	SNACKS AND DESSERT
Day 8 Monday	2 to 4 squares Chocolate-Banana Baked Oatmeal	Leftover Hawaiian Tofu Kabobs Leftover Carrot and Ginger Spiced Rice	Italian Meatballs with Zucchini Noodles Tahini String Beans	**Snacks:** Carrot sticks and hummus Gluten-free pretzels **Dessert:** Dark Chocolate Bark with Pumpkin and Pecans Fruit
Day 9 Tuesday	Breakfast Quinoa	Pantry Bean Soup	Sheet Pan Tilapia and Veggies Broccoli Edamame Salad	**Snacks:** Celery sticks with peanut butter or almond butter Popcorn **Dessert:** Meringue Cookies Fruit
Day 10 Wednesday	2 to 4 squares Chocolate-Banana Baked Oatmeal	Leftover Italian Meatballs with Zucchini Noodles	Roasted Cauliflower and Chickpea Tacos Spinach Strawberry Salad	**Snacks:** Cherry tomatoes Veggie straws **Dessert:** Dark Chocolate Bark with Pumpkin and Pecans Fruit

DAY #	BREAKFAST	LUNCH	DINNER	SNACKS AND DESSERT
Day 11 Thursday	Greek yogurt with fruit and nuts	Mexican Chicken Soup	Beef Tenderloin and Crispy Kale Spiced Peas	**Snacks:** Sliced cucumbers with hummus 2 gluten-free granola bars **Dessert:** Meringue Cookies Fruit
Day 12 Friday	2 to 4 squares Chocolate-Banana Baked Oatmeal	Leftover Roasted Cauliflower and Chickpea Tacos	Turkey Meatball and Kale Soup Fall Carrots and Parsnips	**Snacks:** Mini peppers Potato chips **Dessert:** Chocolate Mousse Fruit
Day 13 Saturday	Avocado Eggs	Mexican Salmon Burgers	Flank Steak "Noodle" Bowls Leftover Spiced Peas	**Snacks:** Celery sticks with peanut butter or almond butter Tortilla chips **Dessert:** Dark Chocolate Bark with Pumpkin and Pecans Fruit
Day 14 Sunday	Blueberry Oat Flour Waffles	Leftover Turkey Meatball and Kale Soup	Spaghetti Squash Lasagna Overnight Marinated Broccoli	**Snacks:** Apple slices 2 gluten-free granola bars **Dessert:** Chocolate Mousse Fruit

LIVING YOUR GLUTEN-FREE LIFE TO THE FULLEST

Congratulations! You've followed this book's meal plan for two weeks and gotten a taste of how delicious the gluten-free lifestyle can be. Shopping for and preparing gluten-free meals should now seem less daunting. To keep your new lifestyle on track, I recommend that you continue creating a shopping list at the beginning of each week, making sure to include a variety of proteins and vegetables so you have flexibility in your meal planning and eating. Don't forget to check on the staples in your pantry, refrigerator, and freezer. If you're low on any items, add them to your shopping list.

Once you have the groceries in your home, you can decide which ingredients to use for which meals during the week (and whether you want or need to prepare anything ahead of time).

You probably noticed that the two-week meal plan contained a wide variety of foods. Try to sustain this variety. Doing so will help you maintain a healthy diet.

When you're outside your home, try to bring along a good cooler and take-out containers to ensure you always have gluten-free food on hand. You may also want to leave portable gluten-free snacks in your car, office, and carry-on bags when you travel. Once you become more familiar with which packaged foods are gluten-free, you'll notice them pretty much everywhere.

If you're just embarking on your gluten-free adventure, know that several months may be needed for your intestines to repair themselves, depending on the severity of the damage. But the human body is quite remarkable: The healing should begin as soon as you cut gluten out of your diet. Of course, if you are not feeling much better after several months, you should absolutely follow up with your doctor. Keep in mind that, once diagnosed, you will probably have regular follow-up appointments throughout the first year. In addition to maintaining a gluten-free diet, regular exercise, sufficient sleep, and proper hydration will help your body repair any damage caused by celiac disease.

A CELIAC'S GUIDE TO EATING OUT

Anyone with celiac disease knows how tricky dining in a restaurant can be, especially somewhere you've never eaten. But provided you avoid the wrong ingredients, ask the right questions, and prepare appropriately, eating out shouldn't be a problem.

It's imperative to avoid soy sauce, teriyaki sauce, salad dressing, and any food-coating sauces when eating out. Critically, many restaurants use something called blended oil to cook their food. This type of oil contains soy sauce, which is not gluten-free.

It is also essential to avoid ordering anything breaded or fried. Although French fries can be made gluten-free when prepared at home from fresh potatoes, most restaurant versions are either coated with gluten to provide a crispy texture or fried in oil with other foods containing gluten. The same goes for fried items like freshly made tortilla chips or potato chips. Food prepared with butter or with nothing else that may contain gluten is okay.

When you are ordering at a restaurant (or for pickup or delivery), alert the wait-staff to your gluten allergy, and ask which food items can be broiled, steamed, or grilled with just non-blended oil and spices. If you desire salad dressing, ask for olive oil and vinegar (or carry a gluten-free dressing with you). You can also order naturally gluten-free side dishes, like vegetables, rice, potatoes, and quinoa, provided they were prepared with no sauces containing gluten.

It's a good idea to call restaurants in advance of a visit to determine whether they are gluten-free friendly. If you are lucky enough to live in a big city, there may be restaurants that are entirely gluten-free.

As for alcoholic drinks, avoid beer and all malt beverages. Distilled liquor is gluten-free because the process of distillation destroys the gluten. However, a problem arises when any flavor is added after the liquor has been distilled, in which case you'll have to review the labels. For the same reason, you should be careful about ordering cocktails. Fortunately, wine is gluten-free and never a problem.

Cross-contamination is another major problem when eating at restaurants, assuming they don't have separate gluten-free kitchens. Utensils like knives, cutting boards, and counters can easily contaminate nearby gluten-free food, and kitchen staff may not know how to keep certain foods gluten-free. Make sure to tell the waitstaff you are allergic to gluten and ask them what the kitchen can do to safely prepare your food for you.

Other environments, such as family gatherings, work events, or birthday parties, can also be troublesome. When in doubt, the best strategy is to bring something along that is gluten-free or stick to eating fresh fruits and vegetables.

Remember, the only way to know for sure whether the food at a restaurant or gathering is gluten-free is to ask. I know how irritating approaching others about gluten content can seem, but when you (or a loved one) has celiac disease, there really isn't any choice. I recommend phrasing questions as follows:

I have celiac disease, which means consuming gluten will make me sick. Do you mind telling me which items on the menu are gluten-free?

If they can't provide a sufficient answer, you may want to be more specific.

To be clear, I can't consume even trace amounts of gluten. Could you tell me what type of oil the restaurant uses to cook its food?

If nothing on the menu is gluten-free, or if the answer to the previous question isn't satisfactory, you might want to say something along the lines of . . .

I apologize for the inconvenience, but could you possibly make something for me without any oil or sauce?

And then list some examples—like rice or vegetables—based on what's on the menu.

When traveling, especially to a foreign country, it's best to choose a hotel that offers rooms with a kitchenette, which will allow you to safely store and prepare gluten-free food. If you are going away for an extended period of time, shipping gluten-free non-perishable foods to your destination may be helpful. Even though many convenience stores and airport concessions sell gluten-free snacks (or alternatives),

I recommend traveling with gluten-free foods in a bag or cooler, so that you always have something available to eat.

WHAT TO DO IF YOU ACCIDENTALLY CONSUME GLUTEN

If you accidentally consume gluten, don't panic. Avoiding all gluten is *incredibly* difficult. All you can do is learn from the experience and try to determine how to prevent future instances. Try to be knowledgeable about which foods to avoid and where to spot hidden sources of gluten (many of which are covered in chapter 2). The symptoms caused by gluten will vary from person to person, but can include gas, bloating, stomach cramps, diarrhea, vomiting, headaches, or a tingling of the extremities. If you believe you've consumed gluten, I recommend following these steps:

1. Determine the offending food or product.

2. Write down how and where you consumed the gluten to avoid the offending food or product in the future.

3. Drink water to prevent dehydration.

4. If you experience the symptoms of dehydration, such as a terrible headache, nausea, or vomiting, seek medical attention.

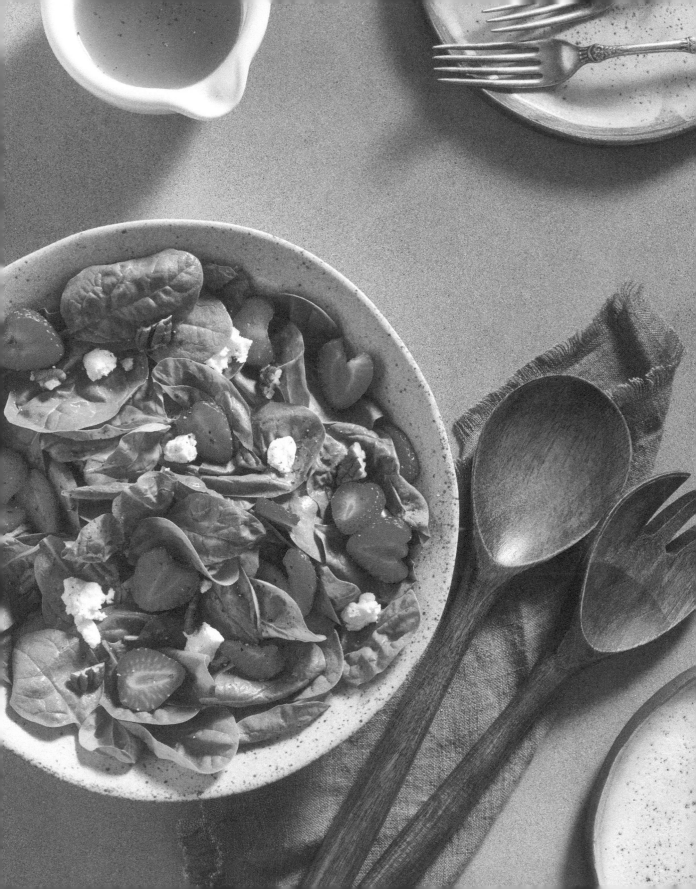

PART TWO

The Recipes

The recipes in this book provide a solid foundation for preparing celiac-friendly food from scratch, so you won't have to rely on highly processed or expensive gluten-free products.

Many of these recipes require only five ingredients—excluding salt, pepper, oil, and vinegar—or take 30 or fewer minutes to make; they are labeled accordingly. My tips will help you avoid cooking mistakes and will help you tweak the recipes on the basis of your preferences or food allergies. Let's get cooking!

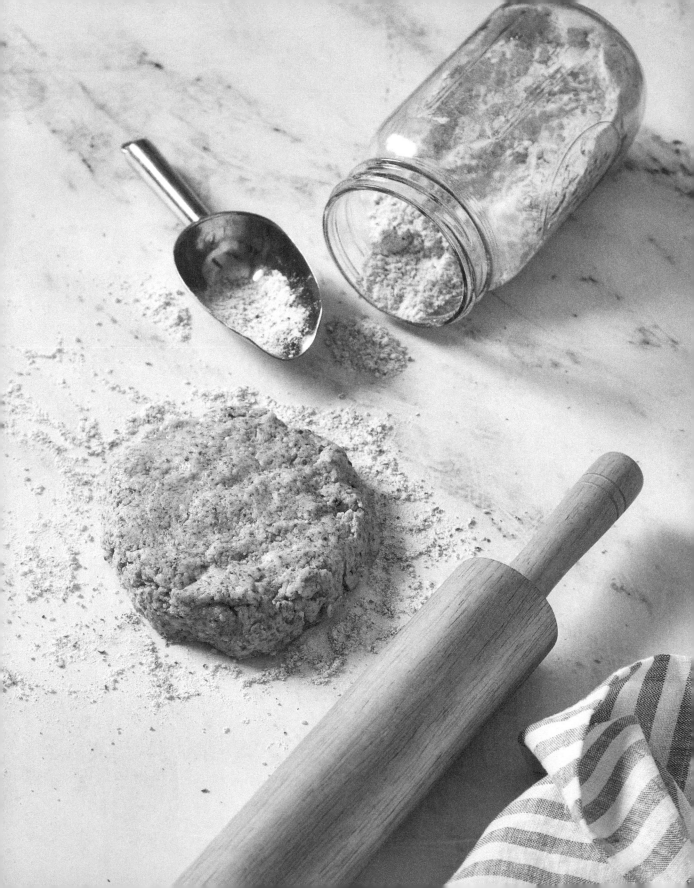

CHAPTER FOUR

The Gluten-Free Essentials

Jamie's All-Purpose Flour Blend

DAIRY-FREE, VEGETARIAN, 30-MINUTE

MAKES 2 CUPS / PREP TIME: 10 MINUTES

With a few batches of my egg-free, all-purpose gluten-free flour blend, you can bake pies, pizzas, and more. Some of the ingredients (sweet rice flour? xanthan gum?) may be unfamiliar to you, but they're all readily available at most supermarkets, often in a devoted gluten-free or health foods section. Bonus: You'll save money by making your flour at home rather than purchasing packaged blends.

¾ cup sweet rice flour

½ cup brown rice flour

¼ cup potato starch

¼ cup tapioca flour

¼ cup almond flour

1 tablespoon xanthan gum

1. In a medium bowl, mix together the sweet rice flour, brown rice flour, potato starch, tapioca flour, almond flour, and xanthan gum.

2. Store in an airtight container in the refrigerator for up to 3 months.

Substitution Tip: If you are allergic to nuts, substitute equal amounts of dry milk powder or soy milk powder for the almond flour.

Per Serving (½ cup): Calories: 309; Saturated Fat: 1g; Total Fat: 5g; Protein: 5g; Total Carbs: 59g; Fiber: 4g; Sodium: 70mg

Jamie's Whole-Grain Flour Blend

DAIRY-FREE, VEGETARIAN, 5-INGREDIENT, 30-MINUTE

MAKES 2 CUPS / PREP TIME: 10 MINUTES

This mixture is a great high-fiber alternative to my All-Purpose Flour Blend. I prefer it for rolls and pizza crusts because the extra fiber contributes to their overall texture and taste. Don't be scared off by the hemp hearts. These nuts are available at most supermarkets.

1 cup brown rice flour

½ cup sweet rice flour

¼ cup ground flaxseed

¼ cup hemp hearts

3 tablespoons xanthan gum

1. In a medium bowl, mix together the brown rice flour, sweet rice flour, ground flaxseed, hemp hearts, and xanthan gum.

2. Store in an airtight container in the refrigerator for up to 3 months.

Substitution Tip: If you prefer, you can swap the hemp hearts for chia seeds. Both of these ingredients increase the fiber content of the flour, which will enhance the texture of your baked goods.

Per Serving (½ cup): Calories: 362; Saturated Fat: 1g; Total Fat: 11g; Protein: 11g; Total Carbs: 56g; Fiber: 13g; Sodium: 198mg

Essential Sandwich Rolls

DAIRY-FREE, VEGETARIAN

MAKES 12 ROLLS / PREP TIME: 20 MINUTES, PLUS 45 MINUTES TO RISE / COOK TIME: 20 MINUTES

These incredibly soft rolls can be prepared with either my all-purpose or whole-grain flour blend. They can be baked in bulk and frozen, so they'll be available whenever you want them.

Nonstick cooking spray

2 cups almond milk

2 (¼-ounce) packets dry yeast

2 teaspoons sugar

3¼ cups Jamie's All-Purpose Flour Blend (page 44)

1 heaping tablespoon baking powder

1 tablespoon xanthan gum

1½ teaspoons salt

2 large eggs, plus 1 large egg

1 teaspoon apple cider vinegar

¼ cup canola oil

¼ cup honey

1. Spray a muffin tin with nonstick cooking spray.

2. In a medium bowl, warm the almond milk in the microwave for 1 minute or in a small pot over low heat for 1 to 2 minutes.

3. Remove the milk from the heat and add the yeast and sugar, mixing well. Set aside for 5 to 10 minutes, until bubbles form.

4. In a large bowl, combine the flour blend, baking powder, xanthan gum, and salt. Add the almond milk mixture, two of the eggs, the vinegar, canola oil, and honey. Using a stand mixer set on the lowest speed, mix the ingredients until just blended. Increase the setting to the highest speed, mixing until a sticky dough forms.

5. Fill each muffin cup two-thirds full.

6. In a small bowl, mix together the remaining egg and a splash of water. Using a small spatula, spread the egg mixture over the top of each unbaked roll.

7. Place the muffin tin in a warm area, such as near the preheating oven, and cover with parchment paper or a clean dishtowel.

8. Wait for the rolls to double in size, about 45 minutes.

9. Preheat the oven to 375°F.

10. When the rolls have doubled in size, uncover and bake for about 20 minutes, or until golden brown.

Substitution Tip: Use my Whole-Grain Flour Blend (page 45) to prepare whole-grain rolls. If you'd prefer, you can also use a packaged gluten-free flour blend, such as King Arthur Flour Measure for Measure, Cup4Cup Multi-Purpose Flour, or Bob's Red Mill 1 to 1.

Per Serving (1 roll): Calories: 304; Saturated Fat: 1g; Total Fat: 8g; Protein: 7g; Total Carbs: 51g; Fiber: 1g; Sodium: 396mg

Essential Pie Crust

VEGETARIAN

MAKES 1 CRUST / PREP TIME: 15 MINUTES, PLUS OVERNIGHT TO SET / COOK TIME: 10 MINUTES, PLUS 15 MINUTES TO COOL

This is my go-to recipe for pie crust. Because it requires time to firm up in the refrigerator, you should always plan to make it a day ahead of time. After the crust is rolled out and baked, use any filling you desire. (See also Very Blueberry Pie, page 129.)

1⅓ cups sweet rice flour

¾ cup almond flour

⅓ cup tapioca flour

¾ cup powdered sugar

3 large eggs

5 tablespoons cold unsalted butter, cut into cubes

¼ cup gluten-free flour, plus more for rolling out dough

1. In a large bowl, combine the sweet rice flour, almond flour, tapioca flour, and powdered sugar. Then add the eggs.

2. Mix in the butter, using two butter knives, until the mixture forms a dough-like consistency.

3. Roll the dough in your hands to form one large ball. Flatten the ball with your hands, forming it into a disc. Wrap the dough in plastic wrap and put it in the refrigerator overnight.

4. When you are ready to bake your crust, preheat the oven to 350°F.

5. Cut two pieces of parchment paper, each about 9 by 13 inches. Place the first piece of parchment on a table and sprinkle it with the gluten-free flour.

6. Unwrap the dough, place it on top of the parchment, and sprinkle with more gluten-free flour. Place the second piece of parchment on top of the dough.

7. Roll out the dough between the two pieces of parchment. Remove the paper and press the dough into a 9-by-13-inch baking dish.

8. Bake for 10 minutes. Let the crust cool for 15 minutes before adding a filling.

Substitution Tip: This recipe can be made dairy-free by substituting equal amounts of margarine for the butter.

Per Serving (⅛ crust): Calories: 488; Saturated Fat: 20g; Total Fat: 35g; Protein: 5g; Total Carbs: 39g; Fiber: 1g; Sodium: 242mg

Essential Pizza Crust

VEGETARIAN

MAKES 1 CRUST / PREP TIME: 15 MINUTES, PLUS 45 MINUTES TO RISE AND 3 HOURS TO CHILL / COOK TIME: 10 MINUTES

Just because you're gluten-free doesn't mean you have to give up pizza. The dough for this delicious crust can be frozen for later use, so consider doubling the recipe. (See page 94 for my favorite pizza recipe.)

1 cup warm water

1 teaspoon sugar

1 (¼-ounce) packet quick-rise yeast

1½ cups Jamie's Whole-Grain Flour Blend (page 45), plus more for rolling out dough

1 tablespoon xanthan gum

1½ teaspoons dry milk powder

1 teaspoon salt

1 tablespoon apple cider vinegar

4 tablespoons olive oil, divided

Make-Ahead Tip: You can freeze the dough for up to a month. When you're ready to use, thaw overnight in the refrigerator or on the counter for a few hours.

Substitution Tip: If you'd prefer to use a store-bought gluten-free flour blend, I would opt for Cup4Cup's wholesome flour blend.

Per Serving (¼ crust): Calories: 264; Saturated Fat: 1g; Total Fat: 12g; Protein: 8g; Total Carbs: 32g; Fiber: 7g; Sodium: 394mg

1. In a medium bowl, combine the water, sugar, and yeast. Set aside to allow bubbles to form, 5 to 10 minutes.

2. Mix in the flour blend, xanthan gum, milk powder, salt, vinegar, and 2 tablespoons of olive oil, until the mixture achieves a dough-like texture.

3. Roll the dough in your hands to form one large ball.

4. Coat the ball of dough with the remaining 2 tablespoons of olive oil.

5. Put the oiled dough back into the bowl, cover, and set aside until it doubles in size, about 45 minutes.

6. After the dough has risen, put it in the refrigerator and chill for 3 hours.

7. Preheat the oven to 400°F.

8. On a flat surface coated with gluten-free flour, roll the dough out until it looks like a flat disc. For easy cleanup, roll it out on floured parchment paper.

9. Place the dough on a sheet pan and bake for 5 to 10 minutes, or until golden brown.

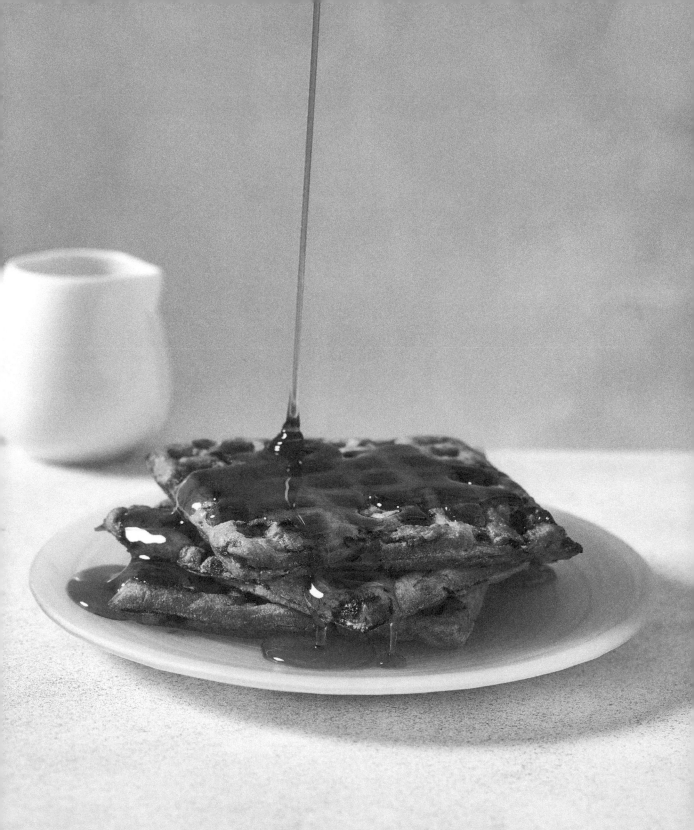

Blueberry Oat Flour Waffles (page 59)

CHAPTER FIVE

Breakfast

Green Eggs and Cheese

VEGETARIAN, 30-MINUTE

SERVES 1 / PREP TIME: 10 MINUTES / COOK TIME: 10 MINUTES

One day after a workout, I went to the kitchen to cook my favorite egg dish—Avocado Eggs (page 55)—and get some good protein and healthy fats. But lo and behold, my kids had eaten the last avocado for breakfast! I took whatever ingredients I could find in my refrigerator—notably, kale, scallions, and feta cheese—and this recipe was born. Now it's one of my absolute favorite breakfasts.

2 teaspoons olive oil

2 scallions, chopped

1 yellow bell pepper, chopped

1 cup chopped fresh kale

½ teaspoon ground cumin

2 large eggs

¼ cup crumbled feta cheese

Salt

Freshly ground black pepper

1. In a medium skillet, heat the oil. Add the scallions and bell pepper, and sauté until softened, 3 to 4 minutes.

2. Mix in the kale and sauté until wilted.

3. Mix in the cumin.

4. With a wooden spoon, create two openings in the pan for the eggs. Crack the eggs into the openings and cook until cooked through, about 3 minutes.

5. Season with salt and pepper, and sprinkle with feta cheese before serving.

Substitution Tip: If you are dairy-free or prefer breakfast meats, you could add cooked sausage as a substitute for the feta cheese.

Per Serving: Calories: 402; Saturated Fat: 10g; Total Fat: 27g; Protein: 21g; Total Carbs: 24g; Fiber: 4g; Sodium: 736mg

Avocado Eggs

DAIRY-FREE, VEGETARIAN, 5-INGREDIENT, 30-MINUTE

SERVES 2 / PREP TIME: 5 MINUTES / COOK TIME: 5 MINUTES

This recipe is a healthier version of eggs in a basket (eggs fried in a hole in a slice of bread). Naturally gluten-free and loaded with healthy fats and fiber, this dish can be topped with Sriracha or another hot sauce of your choice for a little heat before serving.

1 avocado

2 teaspoons avocado oil

2 large eggs

Salt

Freshly ground black pepper

1. Cut the avocado in half, remove the pit and shell, and cut a hole into each half where the pit used to be.
2. In a medium skillet, heat the oil over medium heat. Add the avocado halves, and cook for 1 minute.
3. Crack an egg into the center of each avocado half, and cook to your desired doneness, 3 to 4 minutes.
4. Season to taste with salt and pepper, and serve.

Ingredient Tip: For a heartier meal with more veggies, add chopped tomatoes, onions, and cucumbers on top.

Per Serving: Calories: 247; Saturated Fat: 4g; Total Fat: 22g; Protein: 7g; Total Carbs: 8g; Fiber: 6g; Sodium: 146mg

Mediterranean Egg Cups

VEGETARIAN, 30-MINUTE

MAKES 12 CUPS (6 SERVINGS) / PREP TIME: 10 MINUTES / COOK TIME: 20 MINUTES

This awesome breakfast will transport you, at least for the morning, to the Mediterranean. It is packed with the region's signature ingredients, from olives to feta cheese, and is one of my kids' favorites because it produces 12 muffin-size portions, easily microwaved before school. Don't be afraid to switch up the flavors by tweaking the vegetables and the spices. Alternatively, you could sauté ground turkey and add it to the egg cups before cooking.

Butter, for greasing

8 large eggs

1 tablespoon milk

½ teaspoon dried oregano

Dash salt

Pinch freshly ground black pepper

2 tablespoons diced tomatoes

2 tablespoons sliced Kalamata olives

1 (12-ounce) jar artichoke hearts, drained
   and quartered

1 tablespoon crumbled feta cheese

Sriracha (or hot sauce of your choice),
   for serving

1. Preheat the oven to 350°F.

2. Grease a muffin tin with the butter.

3. In a medium bowl, mix together the eggs, milk, oregano, salt, and pepper.

4. Pour the mixture evenly into each muffin cup.

5. Distribute the tomatoes, olives, and artichoke hearts evenly into each muffin cup.

6. Bake for 15 to 20 minutes, or until the eggs are set.

7. Remove from the oven and top with feta cheese. Serve with Sriracha.

Make-Ahead Tip: Wrap each muffin cup in plastic wrap and freeze them all. You'll have them available to microwave any time you need a quick breakfast.

Per Serving (2 cups): Calories: 137; Saturated Fat: 3g; Total Fat: 9g; Protein: 10g; Total Carbs: 7g; Fiber: 3g; Sodium: 219mg

Breakfast Quinoa

DAIRY-FREE, VEGETARIAN, 5-INGREDIENT

SERVES 2 / PREP TIME: 10 MINUTES / COOK TIME: 20 MINUTES, PLUS 5 MINUTES TO SIT

The first time I tried quinoa for breakfast, I was pretty skeptical. Quinoa can have a bitter taste, and I'd typically only eaten it as part of a savory lunch or dinner. But once I happened upon the right combination of ingredients—those sweet and nutty enough to temper the bitterness—I found this ancient grain extremely satisfying. Doubling or tripling this recipe is also super easy.

1 cup quinoa

2 cups coconut milk

¼ teaspoon salt

¼ cup maple syrup

2 teaspoons almonds, slivered

½ cup raspberries

1. Put the quinoa in a medium bowl; rinse with cold water and drain. Transfer the quinoa to a small saucepan.

2. Mix in the coconut milk and salt, and bring the quinoa to a rolling boil over medium-high heat. Cover the pan, and simmer on low heat for 15 minutes.

3. Turn off the heat and leave the quinoa covered for 5 minutes. Uncover and transfer to two serving bowls.

4. Mix in the maple syrup.

5. Top with almonds and raspberries, and serve.

Ingredient Tip: You can use frozen raspberries here, just be sure to thaw them when you start the recipe.

Per Serving: Calories: 995; Saturated Fat: 51g; Total Fat: 64g; Protein: 18g; Total Carbs: 98g; Fiber: 14g; Sodium: 335mg

Peanut Butter and Jelly Overnight Oats

VEGETARIAN

SERVES 1 / PREP TIME: 15 MINUTES, PLUS OVERNIGHT TO CHILL

There are so many ways to make these oats, and each variation results in an entirely different flavor. This recipe includes my favorite toppings, but feel free to get creative. Try diced apples, pecans, maple syrup, and cinnamon for an apple pie flair. Or, if you're a chocolate person, try maple syrup, almonds, chocolate chips, and shredded coconut. The possibilities are endless!

½ cup rolled old-fashioned gluten-free oats

½ cup milk

¼ cup non-fat plain Greek yogurt

1 tablespoon chia seeds

1 tablespoon honey or maple syrup

¼ teaspoon vanilla extract

¼ cup diced strawberries

2 tablespoons crushed peanuts

1 tablespoon strawberry jam

1 tablespoon peanut butter

1. Put the oats, milk, yogurt, chia seeds, honey, and vanilla in a mason jar. Stir vigorously.

2. Add the strawberries, peanuts, jam, and peanut butter, and stir again.

3. Screw on the lid and put the jar in the refrigerator overnight. For a crunchier texture, add the toppings (strawberries, peanuts, jam, and peanut butter) immediately before serving.

Substitution Tip: To make this recipe dairy-free, substitute almond milk and non-dairy yogurt for the milk and yogurt.

Per Serving: Calories: 657; Saturated Fat: 5g; Total Fat: 27g; Protein: 25g; Total Carbs: 85g; Fiber: 12g; Sodium: 155mg

Blueberry Oat Flour Waffles

DAIRY-FREE, VEGETARIAN, 30-MINUTE

MAKES 6 (3 SERVINGS) / PREP TIME: 15 MINUTES / COOK TIME: 15 MINUTES

Your Sunday brunch is about to get way more interesting. These nutritious blueberry oat waffles are so sweet, you'll have a hard time believing they're gluten-free. Feel free to switch out the blueberries for another seasonal fruit or berry. And if you're feeling particularly decadent, top the waffles with some chocolate chips and whipped cream.

1 cup oat flour

1 tablespoon baking powder

½ cup unsweetened applesauce

¼ cup non-dairy milk

2 tablespoons maple syrup, plus more for serving

1 teaspoon freshly squeezed lemon juice

1 teaspoon vanilla extract

¼ cup fresh or frozen blueberries

Nonstick cooking spray

1. Combine the flour, baking powder, applesauce, milk, maple syrup, lemon juice, and vanilla in a high-speed blender.
2. Blend until combined.
3. Add the blueberries and pulse briefly.
4. Spray a waffle pan or waffle iron with nonstick cooking spray and preheat.
5. Pour some batter into the pan or iron and cook according to the manufacturer's instructions. Repeat with the remaining batter.
6. Serve with maple syrup.

Troubleshooting Tip: If you do not have a waffle pan, spoon the batter into a regular skillet and make blueberry pancakes instead.

Per Serving (2 waffles): Calories: 198; Saturated Fat: 0g; Total Fat: 2g; Protein: 4g; Total Carbs: 40g; Fiber: 4g; Sodium: 38mg

Banana Pancakes

VEGETARIAN, 30-MINUTE

MAKES 12 (4 SERVINGS) / PREP TIME: 10 MINUTES / COOK TIME: 15 MINUTES

These pancakes, with their creamy bananas, are sure to be a crowd-pleaser on lazy weekend mornings. They come together so easily that you won't have to wake up early to prepare them. Just be prepared for your kitchen to smell like a pancake house well into the afternoon—and for whoever sits down at the table to demand seconds.

2 tablespoons unsalted butter

1 cup buckwheat flour

1 teaspoon ground cinnamon

1 teaspoon baking powder

¼ teaspoon salt

3 bananas, mashed

4 large eggs

Maple syrup, for serving

Ingredient Tip: Top these pancakes with extra bananas, almonds, chia seeds, berries, or chocolate chips to change up the taste.

Per Serving (3 pancakes): Calories: 309; Saturated Fat: 4g; Total Fat: 12g; Protein: 12g; Total Carbs: 42g; Fiber: 6g; Sodium: 255mg

1. In a medium skillet, melt the butter over low heat.
2. In a large bowl, mix together the buckwheat flour, cinnamon, baking powder, and salt.
3. In a medium bowl, mash the bananas, then mix in the eggs.
4. Add the banana mixture to the dry ingredients, and mix well.
5. Spoon ⅛ cup batter at a time into the skillet, and cook over medium heat until the pancakes bubble, about 2 minutes. You can cook several pancakes at a time, provided you don't overcrowd the pan.
6. Flip the pancakes, and continue to cook until golden brown. Serve warm with maple syrup.

Chocolate-Banana Baked Oatmeal

DAIRY-FREE, VEGETARIAN

MAKES 12 SQUARES / PREP TIME: 15 MINUTES / COOK TIME: 45 MINUTES

Somewhere between your typical oatmeal and a full-on oatmeal cookie falls baked oatmeal. This particular variation, which brings to mind chocolate chip banana bread, is my personal favorite. This dish delivers all the fiber you'd get from eating regular oatmeal, but it can be prepared ahead of time and stored in the freezer.

Nonstick cooking spray

2 cups gluten-free oats

2 cups water

1 ½ cups almond milk

1 egg

¼ cup chopped peanuts

¼ cup hemp hearts

¼ cup maple syrup

¼ cup peanut butter

1 scoop (1 ½ to 2 tablespoons) gluten-free chocolate protein powder

2 teaspoons ground cinnamon

1 teaspoon vanilla extract

1 ½ whole bananas, plus ½ banana, cut into ¼-inch slices

1. Preheat the oven to 350°F.
2. Spray a 9-by-13-inch baking dish with nonstick cooking spray.
3. In a large bowl, combine the oats, water, milk, egg, peanuts, hemp hearts, maple syrup, peanut butter, protein poweder, cinnamon, vanilla, and the 1½ whole bananas.
4. Distribute the mixture evenly in the baking dish.
5. Top the oatmeal mixture with the remaining banana slices.
6. Bake for 45 minutes, or until golden brown. Cut into 12 equal-size squares before serving.

Ingredient Tip: The chocolate protein powder contributes to the great taste of the oatmeal, and also helps you stay full longer. Quest and Pure Protein both have good gluten-free options.

Per Serving (1 square): Calories: 189; Saturated Fat: 1g; Total Fat: 9g; Protein: 8g; Total Carbs: 21g; Fiber: 4g; Sodium: 98mg

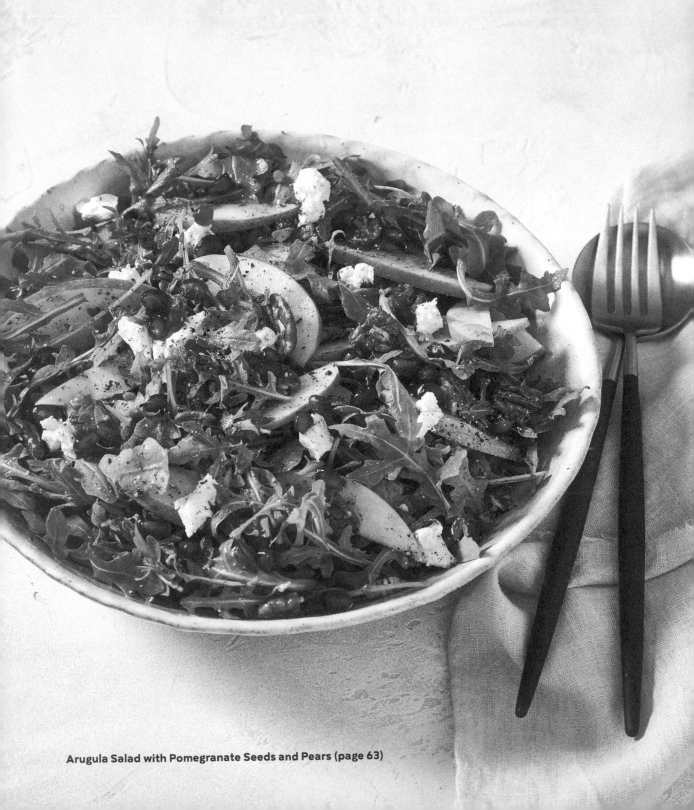

Arugula Salad with Pomegranate Seeds and Pears (page 63)

CHAPTER SIX

Soups, Salads, and Sides

Sweet Red Pepper Gazpacho

DAIRY-FREE, VEGETARIAN, 30-MINUTE

SERVES 4 / PREP TIME: 15 MINUTES

This recipe is most definitely for veggie lovers. There's something so simple and refreshing about a good gazpacho—especially one as attractive as this one, which achieves its vibrant red color from strawberries. For fun, try serving up gazpacho cocktails in fancy martini glasses.

1 cucumber, peeled and chopped

1 tomato, coarsely chopped

1 red bell pepper, coarsely chopped

2 shallots, chopped

1 (1-pound) container strawberries, tops removed

¼ cup vegetable broth

1 tablespoon balsamic vinegar

1 tablespoon freshly squeezed lemon juice

Salt

Freshly ground black pepper

Chopped chives, for garnish

1. Combine the cucumber, tomato, red pepper, shallots, and strawberries in a blender. Blend until smooth.

2. Stir in the broth, vinegar, and lemon juice. Season with salt and pepper.

3. Ladle into bowls, and garnish with chives before serving.

Substitution Tip: If you like a tangier gazpacho, omit the strawberries and add an additional pepper and cucumber.

Per Serving: Calories: 68; Saturated Fat: 0g; Total Fat: 1g; Protein: 2g; Total Carbs: 15g; Fiber: 3g; Sodium: 92mg

Pantry Bean Soup

VEGETARIAN, 30-MINUTE

SERVES 4 / PREP TIME: 10 MINUTES / COOK TIME: 15 MINUTES

Sometimes you just need to make a quick meal from stuff you have in the house. If you're super busy, you'll find this recipe to be a great option because all of the ingredients are probably already sitting right there in your pantry (hence the name). But once you put a dollop of sour cream and scallions on top, the finished product will look like you've worked on it for hours!

2 (15-ounce) cans cannellini beans, rinsed and drained, divided

⅔ cup salsa

1 teaspoon ground cumin

1 teaspoon salt

½ teaspoon freshly ground black pepper

2 cups vegetable stock

Juice of 1 lime

Sour cream, for garnish

Chopped scallions, for garnish

1. Put one can of beans, the salsa, cumin, salt, and pepper into a blender. Blend until smooth, then pour into a medium saucepan.

2. Add the second can of beans, the vegetable stock, and lime juice. Heat over medium-low heat, until the beans are tender.

3. Garnish with sour cream and scallions before serving.

Substitution Tip: Try toasted pumpkin seeds, or even sautéed sausage, as alternative toppings for this soup. And if you're dairy-free, opt for coconut milk instead of sour cream.

Per Serving: Calories: 226; Saturated Fat: 2g; Total Fat: 4g; Protein: 13g; Total Carbs: 37g; Fiber: 11g; Sodium: 543mg

Mexican Chicken Soup

DAIRY-FREE

SERVES 4 / PREP TIME: 10 MINUTES / COOK TIME: 1 HOUR

This recipe is a Mexican-inspired take on a classic chicken soup, and it's just as soulful (but even heartier) with the addition of black beans and roasted tomatoes—not to mention, a bit zestier because of the cumin. You can make this dish in a pot over the stove, but if you have a pressure cooker, now would be a good time to use it.

1 tablespoon olive oil

3 garlic cloves, minced

1 bell pepper, chopped

1 sweet onion, chopped

2 pounds boneless chicken, cut into
    1-inch pieces

1 (15-ounce) can black beans,
    rinsed and drained

1½ cups frozen corn

1 (14.5-ounce) can fire-roasted tomatoes

4 cups chicken broth

2 tablespoons ground cumin

1 teaspoon salt

1. In a large pot, heat the oil over medium heat. Add the garlic, bell pepper, and onion, and cook for 3 minutes, or until the onions are translucent.

2. Add the chicken, black beans, corn, tomatoes, broth, cumin, and salt, and bring to a boil. Cover and simmer for 45 minutes. Place in bowls to serve.

Ingredient Tip: You can garnish this soup with diced scallions, avocado, or even ribbons of zucchini. Alternatively, you could replace half the cumin with a chipotle seasoning, for a spicier dish.

Per Serving: Calories: 476; Saturated Fat: 1g; Total Fat: 9g; Protein: 66g; Total Carbs: 36g; Fiber: 10g; Sodium: 1292mg

Turkey Meatball and Kale Soup

DAIRY-FREE

SERVES 4 / PREP TIME: 30 MINUTES / COOK TIME: 30 MINUTES

Forget chicken noodle: This soup is my go-to comfort food—hearty, rich, and delicious. Plus, the meatballs make this soup satisfying enough to constitute a full meal, particularly if you use my gluten-free Essential Sandwich Rolls (page 46) to soak up the broth. If you're feeling the need for red meat, you can always switch out the ground turkey for ground beef.

For the meatballs

1 pound ground turkey

1 large egg, whipped

3 tablespoons almond flour

2 garlic cloves, crushed

2 tablespoons minced fresh herbs (parsley, basil, dill, or cilantro)

¾ teaspoon salt

½ teaspoon freshly ground black pepper

2 tablespoons coconut oil

For the soup

2 tablespoons coconut oil

1 onion, diced

4 large carrots, chopped

2 garlic cloves, minced

6 cups chicken or vegetable broth

2 dried bay leaves (optional)

1 bunch kale, stemmed and chopped

Chopped fresh herbs (parsley, basil, dill, or cilantro), for garnish

Red pepper flakes, for garnish

To make the meatballs

1. In a large bowl, combine the ground turkey, egg, almond flour, garlic, herbs, salt, and pepper. Mix well.

2. Roll into small balls about 1½ inches in diameter.

3. Heat the coconut oil in a large skillet on medium-high heat.

4. Cook the meatballs for 3 to 4 minutes, until brown. (If all the meatballs don't fit, cook them in batches.) The meatballs will not be cooked through until they are added to the soup.

To make the soup

1. Heat the coconut oil in a large stockpot over medium heat.

2. Add the onions, carrots, and garlic, and cook until the onions are translucent, about 5 minutes.

3. Add the meatballs, broth, and bay leaves (if using). Bring to a boil.

CONTINUED ▶

4. Decrease the heat to low, and simmer for 5 minutes.

5. Add the kale, and cook until the meatballs are cooked through, 5 to 7 minutes.

6. Garnish with fresh herbs and red pepper flakes before serving.

Substitution Tip: If you do not like the flavor of coconut oil, olive oil can be used as a substitute.

Per Serving: Calories: 411; Saturated Fat: 14g; Total Fat: 41g; Protein: 39g; Total Carbs: 19g; Fiber: 4g; Sodium: 788mg

Spinach Strawberry Salad

VEGETARIAN, 30-MINUTE

SERVES 4 / PREP TIME: 15 MINUTES

This salad reminds me of the first days of spring, but I like to serve it all year round. It's incredibly healthy, quick to prepare, and refreshing. You can make the simple dressing ahead of time and keep it in the refrigerator for a few days to use on all your salads.

For the dressing

1 tablespoon balsamic vinegar

¼ tablespoon extra-virgin olive oil

2 teaspoons finely chopped shallots

¼ teaspoon salt

¼ teaspoon freshly ground black pepper

For the salad

6 cups fresh baby spinach

1 cup strawberries, sliced

¼ cup crumbled feta cheese

¼ cup chopped walnuts, toasted

To make the dressing

1. In a large bowl, whisk together the vinegar, oil, shallots, salt, and pepper.

2. If storing for later use, let stand for 5 to 10 minutes, then cover and refrigerate.

To make the salad

1. Put the spinach, strawberries, feta cheese, and walnuts in a large bowl.

2. Add the dressing and toss until the salad is coated before serving.

Substitution Tip: To make this recipe dairy-free, substitute diced avocado for the feta cheese.

Per Serving: Calories: 114; Saturated Fat: 2g; Total Fat: 9g; Protein: 4g; Total Carbs: 6g; Fiber: 2g; Sodium: 288mg

Arugula Salad with Pomegranate Seeds and Pears

VEGETARIAN, 30-MINUTE

SERVES 4 / PREP TIME: 15 MINUTES

This pomegranate and pear-filled garden salad, topped with my favorite ginger dressing, is packed with good-for-you nutrients. The combination of the fruit and goat cheese gently mellows the bitter flavor of the arugula. I recommend using honey crisp apples if they are available. If you don't like arugula, a good substitute would be baby spinach.

For the dressing

¼ cup **extra-virgin olive oil**

1 tablespoon **apple cider vinegar**

1 tablespoon **Dijon mustard**

1 tablespoon **maple syrup or honey**

1 teaspoon **finely grated fresh ginger**

¼ teaspoon **fine sea salt**

Dash **freshly ground black pepper**

For the salad

5 ounces **baby arugula**

½ cup **raw pecans, halved or in pieces**

½ cup **crumbled goat cheese**

1 large **ripe pear, thinly sliced**

1 **apple, thinly sliced**

½ cup **pomegranate seeds**

To make the dressing

In a small bowl, whisk together the oil, vinegar, mustard, maple syrup, ginger, sea salt, and pepper.

To make the salad

1. In a large bowl, mix together the arugula, pecans, goat cheese, pear slices, apple slices, and pomegranate seeds.

2. Toss the salad with dressing just before serving.

Substitution Tip: If you cannot find pomegranate seeds, you can substitute dried cranberries or dried cherries.

Per Serving: Calories: 313; Saturated Fat: 6g; Total Fat: 24g; Protein: 7g; Total Carbs: 22g; Fiber: 4g; Sodium: 222mg

Spicy Cucumber Salad

DAIRY-FREE, VEGETARIAN

SERVES 4, WITH LEFTOVERS / PREP TIME: 10 MINUTES, PLUS 25 MINUTES TO CHILL

Few people can resist a fresh cucumber salad—especially the way I prepare it, with jalepeño, ginger, and dill. Wildly refreshing, this salad has just the right amount of heat. Typically, there aren't any leftovers. But if there are, cover and refrigerate. It will taste even better the next day.

2 large cucumbers, sliced into ¼-inch rounds

¼ cup rice vinegar

2 tablespoons sugar

1 jalapeño pepper, seeded and chopped

½ teaspoon salt

1-inch piece fresh ginger, peeled and chopped

½ teaspoon minced fresh dill

1. Put the sliced cucumbers in a medium glass bowl.

2. In a small bowl, mix together the vinegar, sugar, jalapeño, salt, ginger, and dill.

3. Pour the mixture over the cucumbers and cover with plastic wrap.

4. Chill in the refrigerator for at least 25 minutes before serving.

Per Serving: Calories: 45; Saturated Fat: 0g; Total Fat: 0g; Protein: 1g; Total Carbs: 9g; Fiber: 1g; Sodium: 235mg

Broccoli Edamame Salad

DAIRY-FREE, VEGETARIAN, 30-MINUTE

SERVES 4 / PREP TIME: 15 MINUTES

This Asian-inspired salad is great as a side dish, though you can instantly turn it into the main attraction with the addition of some pre-cooked chicken or tuna. The dressing is a delicious mixture of sweet and savory flavors, like peanut butter and sesame oil, which complement each other perfectly. Here's a hint: The broccoli and edamame mixture is equally delicious over gluten-free or rice noodles, with some chopped peanuts tossed in.

For the dressing

½ cup peanut butter

4 to 5 tablespoons water

2 tablespoons gluten-free soy sauce

2 tablespoons freshly squeezed lime juice

1 tablespoon rice vinegar

1 teaspoon sesame oil

1 teaspoon Sriracha (or hot sauce of your choice)

½ teaspoon honey

½ teaspoon grated ginger

For the salad

1 broccoli head, cut into florets

1 (12-ounce) package fresh or frozen edamame, thawed

3 spring onions, sliced

1 cup salted peanuts

¼ cup sesame seeds

To make the dressing

In a small bowl, mix together the peanut butter, water, soy sauce, lime juice, vinegar, sesame oil, Sriracha, honey, and ginger until combined.

To make the salad

1. In a large bowl, mix together the broccoli, edamame, onions, peanuts, and sesame seeds.

2. Drizzle the dressing over the salad until well coated before serving.

Ingredient Tip: To save time, use pre-cut and bagged broccoli florets.

Per Serving: Calories: 558; Saturated Fat: 9g; Total Fat: 42g; Protein: 28g; Total Carbs: 28g; Fiber: 12g; Sodium: 580mg

Spiced Peas

DAIRY-FREE, VEGETARIAN, 5-INGREDIENT, 30-MINUTE

SERVES 4 / PREP TIME: 5 MINUTES / COOK TIME: 5 MINUTES

If you've avoided peas because your parents made you eat them as a kid, I suggest you try this recipe. These are not your parents' peas! The cumin and red pepper work together to accentuate the fresh, savory flavor of the peas. You can also try puréeing this dish to use as a base beneath a fillet of fish or chicken.

2 teaspoons olive oil

1 teaspoon ground cumin

½ teaspoon red pepper flakes

1 (12-ounce) package fresh or frozen peas, thawed

2 tablespoons chopped fresh parsley

¼ teaspoon salt

1. In a medium skillet, heat the oil over medium heat.

2. Add the cumin and red pepper flakes and stir for a few seconds. Add the peas.

3. Cook for 2 to 3 minutes, or until fresh peas are bright green or frozen peas are heated through.

4. Transfer the peas to a bowl and mix in the parsley and salt before serving.

Substitution Tip: Substitute canned chickpeas as an alternative to the standard peas, if you would like a variation and do not have fresh or frozen peas in your pantry.

Per Serving: Calories: 104; Saturated Fat: 0g; Total Fat: 3g; Protein: 6g; Total Carbs: 15g; Fiber: 5g; Sodium: 154mg

Tahini String Beans

DAIRY-FREE, VEGETARIAN, 5-INGREDIENT, 30-MINUTE

SERVES 4 / PREP TIME: 5 MINUTES / COOK TIME: 10 MINUTES

Tahini, a Mediterranean staple and primary element of hummus, is an underappreciated ingredient that brings out so much flavor in food. In this recipe, this sesame seed-based ingredient is mixed in over hot string beans and tossed with sesame oil for a light, yet satisfying, side.

1 teaspoon olive oil

2 teaspoons sesame oil

1 pound fresh string beans

2 teaspoons gluten-free soy sauce

½ teaspoon freshly ground black pepper

¼ cup tahini

1. In a large skillet, heat the olive oil over medium heat.
2. Add the sesame oil and string beans, and sauté for 2 minutes.
3. Add the soy sauce, pepper, and a splash of water. Cover the skillet and steam the beans for 3 minutes, or until they're bright green.
4. Add the tahini and toss until the beans are coated to serve.

Ingredient Tip: Tahini is readily found in the supermarket and can last for a few months in the refrigerator. The trick is to transfer the tahini to a bowl and give it a stir to reincorporate the separated oils. Return the tahini to its original container once it's combined. You'll want to stir the tahini every time you use it.

Per Serving: Calories: 160; Saturated Fat: 2g; Total Fat: 12g; Protein: 6g; Total Carbs: 12g; Fiber: 5g; Sodium: 494mg

Overnight Marinated Broccoli

DAIRY-FREE, VEGETARIAN, 5-INGREDIENT

SERVES 4 / PREP TIME: 15 MINUTES, PLUS OVERNIGHT TO MARINATE

This recipe is unbelievably easy to prepare, and makes for a reliably palette-pleasing side dish for any dinner. Allowing the broccoli to marinate in a zesty mustard-and-vinegar concoction overnight in the refrigerator softens the broccoli, but leaves all the nutrients intact. If you prefer, use cauliflower florets or a mixture of cauliflower and broccoli.

¼ cup avocado oil

¼ cup apple cider vinegar

3 tablespoons brown sugar

1 tablespoon stone-ground mustard

2 garlic cloves, minced

1 teaspoon salt

¼ teaspoon freshly ground black pepper

2 (12-ounce) bags broccoli florets

1. Put the oil, vinegar, brown sugar, mustard, garlic, salt, and pepper in a large resealable bag.

2. Seal the bag, and squeeze to mix together the ingredients.

3. Add the broccoli to the bag, and reseal.

4. Refrigerate overnight.

5. When you're ready to eat the next day, put the marinated broccoli in a serving bowl and enjoy.

Troubleshooting Tip: If you've got a last-minute dinner to attend and want to bring this dish, but the broccoli hasn't yet marinated overnight—no worries. Though it tastes even better the next day, the vegetable will be marinated enough to enjoy in 2 to 3 hours.

Per Serving: Calories: 216; Saturated Fat: 2g; Total Fat: 15g; Protein: 5g; Total Carbs: 19g; Fiber: 5g; Sodium: 657mg

Fall Carrots and Parsnips

DAIRY-FREE, VEGETARIAN, 5-INGREDIENT

SERVES 4 / PREP TIME: 20 MINUTES / COOK TIME: 35 MINUTES

Roasted carrots are fantastic on their own, but there is something about roasting them with parsnips that makes them extra delicious. The natural bitterness of the parsnips really brings out the sweetness of the carrots. Together, they're the perfect cold-weather side to a meaty entrée.

1 (1-pound) bag carrots, peeled and
    cut into ¼-inch rounds

1 (1-pound) bag parsnips, peeled and
    cut into ¼-inch rounds

2 tablespoons flavor-neutral oil

1 teaspoon salt

½ teaspoon freshly ground black pepper

1. Preheat the oven to 400°F.
2. Put the carrots and parsnips on a sheet pan.
3. Toss with oil, salt, and pepper.
4. Roast for 30 to 35 minutes, or until the vegetables are softened and slightly browned. Serve and enjoy.

Ingredient Tip: You could use baby carrots, but if you do, cut the parsnips into smaller pieces so they are similar in size.

Per Serving: Calories: 192; Saturated Fat: 1g; Total Fat: 7g; Protein: 2g; Total Carbs: 32g; Fiber: 8g; Sodium: 671mg

Healthy Cauliflower Fried Rice

DAIRY-FREE, VEGETARIAN

SERVES 4, WITH LEFTOVERS / PREP TIME: 15 MINUTES / COOK TIME: 30 MINUTES

Sometimes, the best recipes happen by accident. I needed to take a photo of my baked fried rice recipe for a blog post I was writing, but when I went to make a batch for the photo, I discovered I was out of rice. I did have a large bag of riced cauliflower on hand, and figured it would look the same, so I used it instead. Little did I know that the result would be absolutely delicious—not to mention that I could cook it in just a fraction of the time!

Nonstick cooking spray

1 (16-ounce) package frozen
 riced cauliflower

3 tablespoons gluten-free soy sauce

2 tablespoons olive oil

1 red bell pepper, sliced

1 (15-ounce) can baby corn,
 strained and liquid reserved

1 (15-ounce) can bamboo shoots,
 strained and liquid reserved

1 (8-ounce) can water chestnuts,
 strained and liquid reserved

1 (8-ounce) can sliced mushrooms,
 strained and liquid reserved

4 cups liquid (combined reserved
 liquid, plus water)

1. Preheat the oven to 350°F.

2. Lightly coat a 9-by-13-inch baking dish with nonstick cooking spray.

3. In the baking dish, combine the cauliflower, soy sauce, oil, red pepper, baby corn, bamboo shoots, water chestnuts, sliced mushrooms, and the 4 cups of combined reserved liquid.

4. Cover with foil and bake for 30 minutes, or until the water is absorbed. Serve and enjoy.

Substitution Tip: You can use fresh cauliflower instead of the cauliflower rice if you chop the cauliflower into small pieces or pulse in a food processor. If you do, double the baking time to 1 hour.

Per Serving: Calories: 179; Saturated Fat: 1g; Total Fat: 5g; Protein: 7g; Total Carbs: 27g; Fiber: 6g; Sodium: 652mg

Aromatic Vegetable Quinoa

DAIRY-FREE, VEGETARIAN, 5-INGREDIENT

SERVES 4 / PREP TIME: 10 MINUTES / COOK TIME: 30 MINUTES, PLUS 10 MINUTES TO SIT

Quinoa sometimes gets a bad rap because of its bitter taste, but that doesn't have to be the case. Pairing this grain with salt and pepper and aromatics—in this case, fresh carrots and onions—imbues it with great flavor.

1 cup quinoa

2 teaspoons olive oil

1 onion, diced

2 carrots, peeled and chopped

2 celery stalks, chopped

1 teaspoon salt

½ teaspoon freshly ground black pepper

2 cups water

1. Rinse the quinoa in a fine mesh strainer until the water runs clear. Set aside.

2. In a medium saucepan, heat the oil over medium heat. Add the onion, carrots, and celery to the saucepan. Sauté for 2 to 3 minutes, or until the onions are translucent.

3. Add the quinoa, salt, pepper, and water. Bring to a boil.

4. Cover the pan, and simmer over low heat for 15 to 20 minutes, or until all of the water is absorbed.

5. Remove from the heat, and let the quinoa sit covered for 5 to 10 minutes. Fluff with a fork before serving.

Make-Ahead Tip: Rice cookers work very well for quinoa. The cooking process will take longer, but you can set it and forget it. Use the mixed rice setting. Sauté the veggies, add them to the quinoa, and serve.

Per Serving: Calories: 202; Saturated Fat: 1g; Total Fat: 5g; Protein: 7g; Total Carbs: 33g; Fiber: 5g; Sodium: 613mg

Carrot and Ginger Spiced Rice

DAIRY-FREE, VEGETARIAN, 5-INGREDIENT

SERVES 4 / PREP TIME: 10 MINUTES / COOK TIME: 30 MINUTES, PLUS 30 MINUTES TO SIT

This recipe makes it surprisingly easy to infuse your basmati rice with an intense Indian-inspired flavor. The combination of onion, carrots, ginger, and salt does the trick. And there's a bonus: This spiced rice is amazingly fluffy every time. You may never be satisfied with standard basmati rice ever again!

2 cups basmati rice

2 teaspoons flavor-neutral oil

1 onion, diced

1 (10-ounce) bag shredded carrots

1-inch piece fresh ginger, peeled and minced

1 teaspoon salt

4 cups water

1. Rinse the rice in a bowl under cold water until the water runs clear. Set aside.

2. In a medium pot, heat the oil over medium heat.

3. Add the onion, and sauté for 2 to 3 minutes, or until translucent.

4. Add the carrots, ginger, and rice. Toss until coated with oil.

5. Add the salt and water, then increase the heat to medium-high and cook until about 90 percent of the water is absorbed.

6. Cover the pot, and simmer on low heat for 10 minutes.

7. Turn off the heat, and leave the pot covered for 30 minutes. Fluff with a fork before serving.

Substitution Tip: You can substitute any other vegetables you like as long as they are diced into small pieces.

Per Serving: Calories: 398; Saturated Fat: 1g; Total Fat: 3g; Protein: 8g; Total Carbs: 84g; Fiber: 4g; Sodium: 636mg

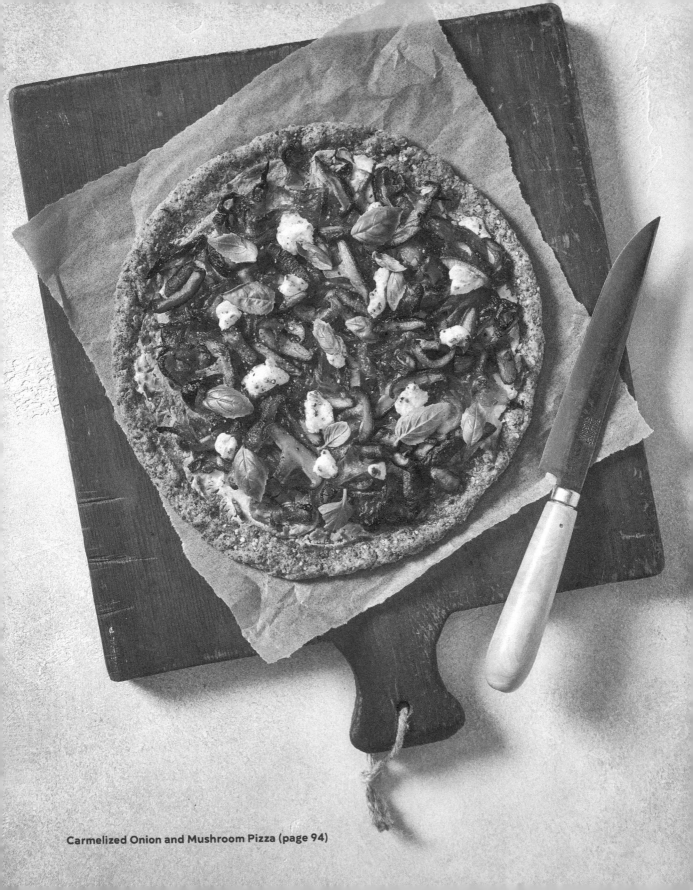

Carmelized Onion and Mushroom Pizza (page 94)

Meatless Mains

Quinoa Stuffed Peppers

DAIRY-FREE, VEGETARIAN

MAKES 6 (4 SERVINGS) / PREP TIME: 15 MINUTES / COOK TIME: 55 MINUTES, PLUS 5 MINUTES TO REST

These protein-packed stuffed peppers are a great weekend lunch or weeknight dinner idea. They're filling, healthy, and surprisingly easy to make. For an even heartier twist, sauté some canned beans with the onions, and use them as extra stuffing, in addition to the quinoa.

Nonstick cooking spray

½ cup tri-color quinoa

1 cup water

2 tablespoons coconut oil

1 carrot, peeled and diced

½ small onion, diced

1 (12-ounce) package firm tofu, diced

3 garlic cloves, minced

Salt

Freshly ground black pepper

6 yellow bell peppers

1. Preheat the oven to 350°F.

2. Grease a 9-by-13-inch baking dish with nonstick cooking spray.

3. Rinse the quinoa in a fine mesh strainer until the water runs clear. Put the quinoa in a small saucepan and add the water. Boil about 10 minutes, or until the water is absorbed. Turn off the heat, and cover the saucepan.

4. In a large skillet, heat the coconut oil over medium-high heat. Add the carrot, onion, tofu, and garlic. Sauté for about 5 minutes, or until the vegetables are soft. Season generously with salt and pepper.

5. Increase the heat to high, add the cooked quinoa, and stir for an additional 1 to 2 minutes. Remove from the heat.

6. Cut off the pepper tops and remove the seeds. Spoon the quinoa and vegetable mixture into the peppers.

7. Place the stuffed peppers into the prepared baking dish and bake for 25 to 30 minutes, or until the peppers are softened but not mushy.

8. Remove the stuffed peppers from the oven, and let sit for 5 minutes before serving.

Make-Ahead Tip: You can prepare the quinoa by cooking it in advance and storing it covered in the refrigerator. You can also prep the peppers in advance to save time. Just keep them covered separately in the refrigerator.

Per Serving (1½ peppers): Calories: 268; Saturated Fat: 6g; Total Fat: 12g; Protein: 12g; Total Carbs: 33g; Fiber: 6g; Sodium: 66mg

Hawaiian Tofu Kabobs

DAIRY-FREE, VEGETARIAN, 5-INGREDIENT

SERVES 4 / PREP TIME: 15 MINUTES, PLUS 1 HOUR TO MARINATE / COOK TIME: 15 MINUTES

Tofu is easy to prepare and surprisingly tasty because it absorbs the flavors of whatever you cook it with—in this case, a slightly sweet, Hawaiian-inspired marinade made with gluten-free hoisin sauce. With the addition of peppers and pineapple, this inventively tropical dish will be a pleasure to share with your family and friends.

1 (12-ounce) package firm tofu

2 red bell peppers, sliced

1 (20-ounce) can pineapple chunks

1 (10-ounce) jar gluten-free hoisin sauce

¼ cup sesame oil

Troubleshooting Tip: If you do not have metal skewers, you can make this dish just by cooking the ingredients together on a sheet pan or, alternatively, by sautéing them all in a wok.

Per Serving: Calories: 431; Saturated Fat: 3g; Total Fat: 20g; Protein: 11g; Total Carbs: 57g; Fiber: 6g; Sodium: 1158mg

1. Cut the tofu into large chunks, and put them into a medium bowl.

2. Put the peppers and pineapple in a separate medium bowl.

3. In a small bowl, mix the hoisin and sesame oil. Pour half of the mixture over the tofu and half over the pineapple and peppers, tossing to coat the ingredients with the sauce. Cover the bowls, and put them in the refrigerator.

4. Marinate for at least 1 hour.

5. Preheat the oven to 425°F.

6. To make the kabobs, alternate ingredients on metal skewers and place on a parchment-lined sheet pan.

7. Bake for 15 minutes. Serve warm.

Avocado Cilantro Enchiladas

DAIRY-FREE, VEGETARIAN

MAKES 6 ENCHILADAS / PREP TIME: 20 MINUTES / COOK TIME: 50 MINUTES

Mexican restaurants may be difficult to negotiate if you have celiac disease, but there's no reason you can't enjoy delicious Mexican food at home. I know the instructions may look daunting, but don't be intimidated. These enchiladas are deceptively easy to make. Plus, after you've made my avocado cilantro sauce, you'll want to drizzle it over everything. Tasty topping ideas for this dish include cilantro, jalapeños, and avocado slices.

For the avocado cilantro sauce

2 tablespoons olive oil

½ red onion, coarsely chopped

2 garlic cloves, coarsely chopped

1½ teaspoons ground cumin

Dash salt

½ avocado

½ bunch cilantro, with stems

¼ cup water

For the enchiladas

½ head cauliflower, coarsely chopped

2 teaspoons avocado oil

½ red onion, diced

1 red bell pepper, diced

1 (15-ounce) can black beans, rinsed and drained

1½ teaspoons ground cumin

Dash salt

1½ cups red enchilada sauce, divided

8 corn tortillas

To make the avocado cilantro sauce

1. In a small saucepan, heat the olive oil over medium heat.

2. Add the onion, garlic, cumin, and salt.

3. Sauté for about 5 minutes, or until the onions begin to soften.

4. Put the onion mixture, avocado, cilantro, and water into a blender.

5. Blend on high until combined.

6. Pour into a bowl and set aside.

To make the enchiladas

1. Add the cauliflower to a medium pot and cover with water.

2. Bring to a boil over high heat, then simmer for about 10 minutes, or until the cauliflower is fork tender. Drain the cauliflower, transfer to a small bowl, and set aside.

3. In a medium skillet, heat the avocado oil over medium heat.

CONTINUED ▶

4. Add the onion, bell pepper, black beans, cumin, salt, and ¼ cup of enchilada sauce to the skillet. Sauté for 5 to 7 minutes, or until the onions and bell pepper are softened.

5. Place the pot used to simmer the cauliflower back on the stove. Put the drained cauliflower, half the avocado cilantro sauce, and ¼ cup of enchilada sauce into the pot.

6. Using a potato masher or wooden spoon, break apart the cauliflower until it is fully combined with the enchilada sauce. Add the onion, bell pepper, and bean mixture to the cauliflower, and stir to combine.

7. Preheat the oven to 350°F.

8. Wrap the tortillas in a damp paper towel and steam in the microwave for 30 seconds.

9. Cover the bottom of a 9-by-13-inch baking dish with ½ cup of enchilada sauce.

10. Fill each tortilla with about ¼ cup of the mixture, then roll them up.

11. Place each filled tortilla seam-side down in the baking dish.

12. Top with the remaining ½ cup of enchilada sauce, and bake in the oven for 20 minutes.

13. Serve with remaining avocado cilantro sauce.

Ingredient Tip: Enchilada sauce can be purchased in a jar in most supermarkets. It's also sold in packets, which you can mix with water to make the sauce.

Per Serving (1 enchilada): Calories: 223; Saturated Fat: 1g; Total Fat: 8g; Protein: 7g; Total Carbs: 34g; Fiber: 9g; Sodium: 421mg

Roasted Cauliflower and Chickpea Tacos

DAIRY-FREE, VEGETARIAN, 30-MINUTE

SERVES 4 / PREP TIME: 25 MINUTES / COOK TIME: 5 MINUTES

These tacos are terrific for a weeknight, especially if you make a habit of keeping some frozen cauliflower in the freezer. They're satisfyingly meaty—without any actual meat, of course. To keep things interesting from one taco night to the next, try switching up the toppings: Sour cream, spicy mayo, diced avocado, and/or a simple coleslaw all work great. This recipe calls for Sriracha, but feel free to use the hot sauce of your choice!

1 (14-ounce) package frozen cauliflower, cut into bite-size pieces

1 (15-ounce) can chickpeas, strained and liquid reserved, divided

2 tablespoons Sriracha

2 tablespoons apple cider vinegar

1 tablespoon tomato paste

1 tablespoon Dijon mustard

2 teaspoons olive oil

1 carrot, peeled and chopped

2 to 4 garlic cloves, minced

1 celery stalk, chopped

1 small onion, chopped

Salt

Freshly ground black pepper

8 corn tortillas or taco shells, or more as needed

1. Put the frozen cauliflower in a strainer in the sink. Run cold water over the cauliflower to defrost.

2. In a small bowl, whisk together ¼ cup of reserved chickpea liquid with the Sriracha, vinegar, tomato paste, and mustard.

3. In a separate small bowl, mash ½ cup of chickpeas.

4. Add the seasoned liquid to the mashed chickpeas. Set aside.

5. In a large skillet, heat the oil over medium heat. Add the carrot, garlic, celery, and onion. Sauté for about 3 minutes, or until the vegetables are softened.

6. Add the mashed chickpea mixture and the remaining chickpeas to the skillet. Stir for about 1 minute, or until they're heated through.

CONTINUED ▶

7. Turn off the heat. Season with salt and pepper.

8. Layer the mixture inside corn tortillas or taco shells, and top as desired.

Troubleshooting Tip: If you find that the vegetables stick to the pan, slowly add small amounts of the reserved liquid from the chickpeas.

Per Serving: Calories: 229; Saturated Fat: 1g; Total Fat: 5g; Protein: 10g; Total Carbs: 39g; Fiber: 10g; Sodium: 161mg

Chickpea Curry with Kale

DAIRY-FREE, VEGETARIAN

SERVES 4 / PREP TIME: 10 MINUTES / COOK TIME: 35 MINUTES

Even if you aren't a fan of curry, I'm confident this dish will win you over. The freshness of the ginger really brings out the flavors of the curry spice blend, which is all wonderfully absorbed by the chickpeas and the kale. To make this meal more substantial, serve over the rice of your choice (I actually prefer cauliflower rice).

For the spice blend

1 teaspoon ground cumin

1 teaspoon ground turmeric

1 teaspoon ground coriander

1 teaspoon sea salt

½ teaspoon cayenne pepper

For the curry

1 teaspoon coconut oil

1 small red onion, finely chopped

1 medium sweet potato, diced

2 garlic cloves, minced

1-inch piece fresh ginger, peeled and minced

1 (8-ounce) can diced tomatoes

½ cup vegetable stock or water

½ cup full-fat coconut cream, separated from the coconut milk

2 (15.5-ounce) cans chickpeas, rinsed and drained

3 cups stemmed and chopped fresh kale

To make the spice blend

In a small bowl, combine the cumin, turmeric, coriander, salt, and cayenne pepper. Mix well.

To make the curry

1. In a large skillet, heat the oil over medium heat.

2. Add the onion and cook for 2 to 3 minutes, or until fragrant and translucent.

3. Stir in the sweet potato and cook for another 2 minutes.

4. Add the garlic, ginger, and spice blend, and cook for another 30 seconds.

5. Add the tomatoes with their juices, stock, and coconut cream, then stir to combine.

6. Cover and cook over high heat, bringing the curry to a low boil. Add the chickpeas, then reduce the heat to low and simmer for about 20 minutes, or until the sweet potato is tender.

CONTINUED ▶

7. Remove from the heat and stir in the kale before serving.

Ingredient Tip: Refrigerate a can of coconut milk overnight to more effectively separate the cream. The next day, the cream will have risen to the top of the can.

Per Serving: Calories: 361; Saturated Fat: 8g; Total Fat: 12g; Protein: 15g; Total Carbs: 53g; Fiber: 13g; Sodium: 520mg

Spaghetti Squash Lasagna

VEGETARIAN

SERVES 4 / PREP TIME: 20 MINUTES / COOK TIME: 40 MINUTES

This recipe is just as delicious as a traditional lasagna or baked ziti, but much healthier and lower in calories. Although spaghetti squash can seem intimidating, they are easy to prepare. Just don't expect leftovers: You can rest assured this dish will be gobbled up in one sitting.

4 spaghetti squash

1 large egg

1 teaspoon dried oregano

Dash salt

Dash freshly ground black pepper

9 ounces fresh baby spinach

1 (16-ounce) jar marinara sauce

1 (8-ounce) package shredded mozzarella cheese

1. Preheat the oven to 350°F.
2. Prick each spaghetti squash all around with a fork.
3. Microwave each squash on high for 10 minutes.
4. When cool enough to touch, slice the spaghetti squash in half, remove the seeds, and scoop out the squash into a large bowl.
5. Add the egg, oregano, salt, and pepper to the squash, and mix well.
6. Spread the squash mixture evenly across a 9-by-13-inch baking dish.
7. Spread an even layer of spinach on top of the squash mixture. Spread the marinara sauce in an even layer over the spinach. Top with mozzarella cheese.
8. Bake for 30 minutes, or until the cheese is bubbling and melted. Serve warm.

Troubleshooting Tip: If you do not have a microwave, you can prepare the squash by slicing it in half, drizzling it with a little oil, placing it cut-side down on a sheet pan, and roasting it in the oven for 45 minutes at 350°F.

Per Serving: Calories: 335; Saturated Fat: 6g; Total Fat: 12g; Protein: 15g; Total Carbs: 50g; Fiber: 1g; Sodium: 456mg

Red Bean and Quinoa Burgers

DAIRY-FREE, VEGETARIAN

MAKES 6 BURGERS / PREP TIME: 15 MINUTES / COOK TIME: 30 MINUTES

Who needs meat when you've got homemade veggie burgers this delicious? Prepackaged veggie burgers can be dry and tasteless, but these burgers stay moist and tender because they're made by mixing fresh quinoa with mashed beans. The combination results in a satisfyingly tender patty. I recommend making extra and freezing the leftovers for a quick lunch or dinner. These burgers would also be terrific served either over a salad or on my Essential Sandwich Rolls (page 46).

1 cup quinoa

2 cups water

2 (15-ounce) cans red beans, rinsed and drained

½ cup mayonnaise

3 scallions, chopped

1 teaspoon ground cumin

½ teaspoon salt

¼ teaspoon freshly ground black pepper

⅓ cup chickpea flour

2 tablespoons flavor-neutral oil

Ingredient Tip: Sliced avocado, sliced tomatoes, and sautéed mushrooms make great toppings for these burgers.

Per Serving (1 burger): Calories: 360; Saturated Fat: 2g; Total Fat: 16g; Protein: 13g; Total Carbs: 42g; Fiber: 9g; Sodium: 322mg

1. Rinse the quinoa in a fine mesh strainer until the water runs clear.

2. Put the quinoa in a small saucepan and add the water. Bring to a boil over high heat, then cover. Cook over low heat, simmering for about 15 minutes, or until the water is absorbed. Set aside.

3. In a large bowl, mash the beans with a fork. Add the mayonnaise, scallions, cumin, salt, and pepper. Mix until smooth.

4. Add the cooked quinoa and the chickpea flour. Mix until combined.

5. Divide the mixture into six equal portions, then form them into patties with your hands.

6. Heat the oil in a large skillet over medium-high heat. Without overcrowding the pan, cook the burgers for 4 minutes on each side, or until golden brown. Serve and enjoy.

Portobello Mushroom Pizza

VEGETARIAN, 5-INGREDIENT, 30-MINUTE

MAKES 4 PIZZAS (2 SERVINGS) / PREP TIME: 5 MINUTES / COOK TIME: 10 MINUTES, PLUS 5 MINUTES TO COOL

Good news: Pizza isn't off-limits just because you're gluten-free. And it doesn't always have to be as complicated as preparing a gluten-free crust. My daughter loves this healthy iteration, which is made with tasty portobello mushroom caps as the base. The quick preparation time makes this dish a great afternoon (or even late-night) snack.

4 portobello mushroom caps

¼ cup marinara sauce, divided

4 dashes Italian seasoning, divided

1 cup shredded mozzarella cheese, divided

1. Preheat the oven to 400°F.

2. Place the mushroom caps top down on a sheet pan lined with parchment paper.

3. Top each mushroom cap with marinara sauce.

4. Top each cap with a dash of Italian seasoning.

5. Sprinkle shredded mozzarella cheese evenly over each cap.

6. Bake for about 10 minutes, or until the cheese is melted and bubbling.

7. Allow to cool for 5 minutes before serving.

Substitution Tip: Switch it up by using slices of zucchini or eggplant instead of portobello mushrooms. If using eggplant, slice it very thin or precook slices before topping them.

Per Serving (2 mushrooms): Calories: 216; Saturated Fat: 8g; Total Fat: 10g; Protein: 18g; Total Carbs: 14g; Fiber: 4g; Sodium: 532mg

Caramelized Onion and Mushroom Pizza

VEGETARIAN, 5-INGREDIENT

SERVES 4 / PREP TIME: 10 MINUTES / COOK TIME: 1 HOUR

For a gourmet flair, sautéed mushrooms and onions are strewn over this delicious pizza. Be sure to drizzle the honey on liberally before serving to bring out the sweetness of the onions.

1 Essential Pizza Crust (page 50)

Olive oil, for greasing

2 (8-ounce) boxes shiitake mushrooms, chopped

4 sweet onions, thinly sliced

1 (4-ounce) package goat cheese

3 tablespoons honey

Substitution Tip: If you want to make this recipe dairy-free, you can spread a thin layer of tomato sauce instead of the cheese.

Per Serving: Calories: 493; Saturated Fat: 5g; Total Fat: 18g; Protein: 16g; Total Carbs: 71g; Fiber: 12g; Sodium: 694mg

1. Preheat the oven to 400°F

2. Bake the crust for 10 minutes on a pizza stone or sheet pan, then set aside to cool.

3. While the crust is baking, grease a small skillet, and put the chopped mushrooms into the skillet. Sauté over medium heat for 10 minutes, or until softened.

4. Add the sliced onions, and sauté for 5 minutes more, or until the onions begin to brown. Add a splash of water, and continue to sauté until the onions are caramelized. They will be very soft and golden brown.

5. Spread the goat cheese over the cooled pizza crust. Layer the mushrooms and onions on top. Drizzle with honey.

6. Bake for 20 minutes, or until the crust is golden and the cheese is bubbling. Serve warm.

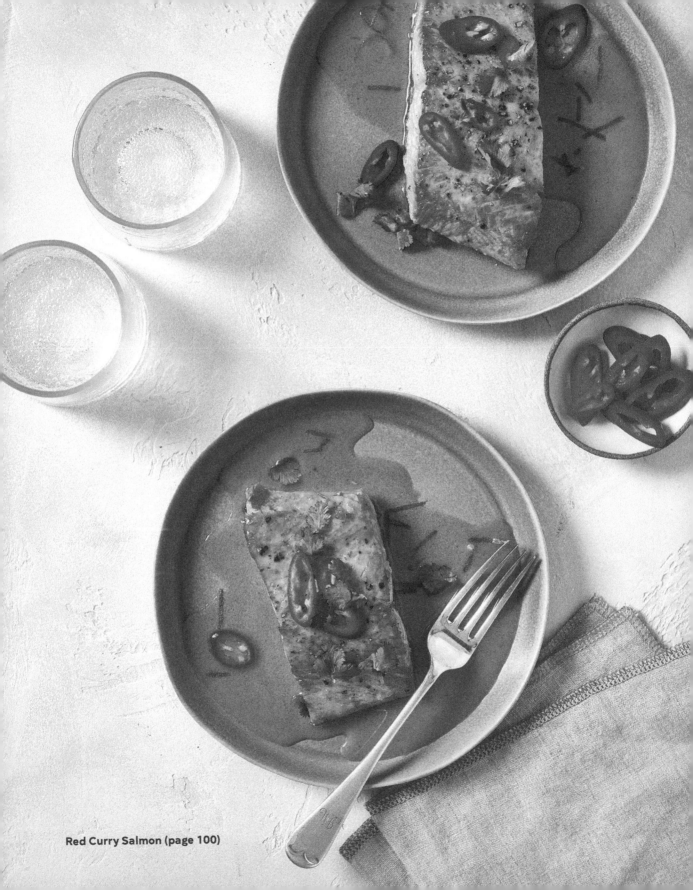

Red Curry Salmon (page 100)

Fish and Seafood

Sheet Pan Tilapia and Veggies

DAIRY-FREE, 30-MINUTE

SERVES 4 / PREP TIME: 15 MINUTES / COOK TIME: 15 MINUTES

Simple sheet pan meals yield consistently great results, even when you switch up the ingredients. This one, made with tilapia, asparagus, broccoli, and Mediterranean-inspired spices, exhibits a particularly harmonious balance of flavors—and can be cooked very quickly. In just 30 minutes, you'll have a full meal for your family to enjoy (or a few days' worth of lunches for yourself).

4 (6-ounce) tilapia fillets

1 large zucchini, sliced

2 cups broccoli florets

1 bunch asparagus, ends trimmed

1 pint cherry tomatoes

2 garlic cloves, crushed and diced

3 tablespoons olive oil

2 tablespoons freshly squeezed
   lemon juice

1 tablespoon chopped fresh parsley

1 teaspoon dried oregano

Dash salt

Pinch freshly ground black pepper

1. Preheat the oven to 400°F.

2. Arrange the tilapia, zucchini, broccoli, asparagus, and tomatoes on a sheet pan.

3. In a small bowl, mix the garlic, olive oil, lemon juice, parsley, oregano, salt, and pepper.

4. Drizzle the oil mixture over the fish and vegetables, tossing to coat.

5. Bake for 12 to 15 minutes, or until the fish flakes with a fork. Serve warm.

Substitution Tip: If you do not enjoy tilapia, other fish like Chilean sea bass, red snapper, salmon, or halibut could work equally as well in this dish.

Per Serving: Calories: 290; Saturated Fat: 2g; Total Fat: 13g; Protein: 36g; Total Carbs: 12g; Fiber: 4g; Sodium: 130mg

Mexican Salmon Burgers

DAIRY-FREE, 30-MINUTE

SERVES 4 / PREP TIME: 20 MINUTES / COOK TIME: 10 MINUTES

Eat these burgers as is or serve them on my Essential Sandwich Rolls (page 46). Either way, top them with generous amounts of my creamy avocado salsa.

For the burgers

4 (¼-pound) salmon fillets, skinned
  and chopped

½ cup almond flour

1 large egg

2 scallions, chopped

½ poblano pepper, seeded and chopped

1 tablespoon freshly squeezed
  lemon or lime juice

½ teaspoon salt

¼ teaspoon freshly ground black pepper

For the avocado salsa

1 large ripe avocado, chopped

½ poblano pepper, seeded and chopped

2 scallions, chopped

1 tablespoon freshly squeezed lemon juice

¼ teaspoon salt

¼ teaspoon freshly ground black pepper

Substitution Tip: You can make this recipe with canned salmon to save time.

Per Serving: Calories: 339; Saturated Fat: 4g; Total Fat: 23g; Protein: 26g; Total Carbs: 7g; Fiber: 4g; Sodium: 527mg

To make the burgers

1. Put the chopped salmon into a large bowl.

2. Add the almond flour, egg, scallions, poblano pepper, lemon juice, salt, and pepper to the salmon, and mix well.

3. Form the salmon mixture into 4 patties.

4. Heat an indoor grill pan or outdoor grill to medium-high heat.

5. Cook each burger about 4 minutes on each side, or until cooked through.

6. Top the burgers with salsa before serving.

To make the avocado salsa

In a medium bowl, add the avocado, poblano pepper, scallions, lemon juice, salt, and pepper. Mix well. Set aside on the counter if using within 30 minutes. Store covered in the refrigerator if you are preparing it ahead of time.

Red Curry Salmon

DAIRY-FREE, 30-MINUTE

SERVES 4 / PREP TIME: 10 MINUTES / COOK TIME: 15 MINUTES

The flavors from this delicious dish take their cues from a traditional Thai red curry, but they are mild enough for everyone to enjoy. The secret is the smooth, caramelized coconut lime sauce, made with lemongrass, ginger, and chili garlic paste. For extra credit, you can serve this dish over rice noodles or steamed vegetables (try bok choy!).

4 (6-ounce) salmon fillets

Salt

Freshly ground black pepper

2 tablespoons avocado oil, divided

2 garlic cloves, finely minced

2 teaspoons finely grated fresh ginger

1 lemongrass stalk, peeled and finely grated

1 tablespoon brown sugar

1 tablespoon tamari

1 teaspoon chili garlic paste

1 (14-ounce) can coconut milk

2 teaspoons grated lime zest

Lime juice

Fresh cilantro leaves, finely chopped, for garnish (optional)

Large red chiles, finely sliced, for garnish (optional)

1. Season the salmon with salt and pepper.

2. In a large skillet, heat 1 tablespoon of oil over medium-high heat.

3. Add the salmon, skin-side up, and sear for 1½ minutes, or until golden.

4. Turn the salmon over, and cook the other side for 1 minute. Remove the salmon from the heat and transfer the fillets to a plate (the salmon should still be raw inside). Decrease the heat to medium-low and allow the skillet to cool.

5. In the same skillet, heat the remaining 1 tablespoon of oil. Add the garlic, ginger, and lemongrass. Cook about 1 minute, or until the garlic is light golden brown.

6. Add the brown sugar and cook for 20 seconds, or until the mixture becomes a caramel color. Stir in the tamari and chili garlic paste.

7. Add the coconut milk and stir, scraping the skillet to dissolve any bits stuck on the bottom. Increase the heat to medium. Simmer for 2 minutes.

8. Place the salmon into the sauce, lower the heat, and gently simmer for 4 minutes, or until the salmon is cooked through.

9. Remove the salmon, and stir in the lime zest and juice to taste.

10. Spoon additional sauce over the salmon, and garnish with cilantro and chiles (if using) before serving.

Ingredient Tip: Chili garlic paste is great for seasoning food; it also works well as a topping and dipping sauce. You can find it in the Asian section of the supermarket.

Per Serving: Calories: 605; Saturated Fat: 26g; Total Fat: 48g; Protein: 36g; Total Carbs: 9g; Fiber: 3g; Sodium: 404mg

Sriracha Fish Tacos

DAIRY-FREE, 30-MINUTE

SERVES 4 / PREP TIME: 10 MINUTES / COOK TIME: 15 MINUTES

Who doesn't love fish tacos? These are super easy to whip up anytime of the week. The spicy homemade Sriracha mayo is a must if you want to intensify the flavor, whereas the shredded cabbage cools everything down. If you want a lighter version, you could wrap the tacos with lettuce leaves instead of tortillas.

For the fish tacos

3 large eggs

1 cup apple cider

1½ cups cornmeal

1 tablespoon chili powder

2 teaspoons dry mustard powder

1 teaspoon salt

¼ cup olive oil

1½ pounds cod, cut into about 12 strips

8 corn tortillas

1 cup shredded cabbage

For the Sriracha mayo

1 cup mayonnaise

1 tablespoon Sriracha (or hot sauce of your choice)

Juice of ½ lime

1 to 2 tablespoons chopped cilantro

To make the fish tacos

1. In a medium bowl, mix together the eggs, apple cider, cornmeal, chili powder, mustard powder, and salt.

2. Line a plate with paper towels and set aside.

3. In a large skillet, heat the oil over medium-high heat.

4. Dip each strip of cod into the batter (there should be about 12 strips).

5. Fry each strip in the oil for 5 minutes on each side, or until browned and cooked through. Transfer the fried fish to the lined plate.

6. Place 1 or 2 pieces of fried fish into each tortilla. Top with Sriracha mayo and cabbage to serve.

To make the Sriracha mayo

In a medium bowl, combine the mayonnaise, Sriracha, lime juice, and cilantro. Mix well. You can store leftover spicy mayo in an airtight container in the refrigerator for up to a week.

Ingredient Tip: Chopped scallions, diced tomatoes, and diced avocado make great additional toppings.

Per Serving: Calories: 983; Saturated Fat: 10g; Total Fat: 63g; Protein: 42g; Total Carbs: 68g; Fiber: 8g; Sodium: 1181mg

Maple-Ginger Red Snapper

DAIRY-FREE

SERVES 4 / PREP TIME: 10 MINUTES / COOK TIME: 30 MINUTES

Packed with vitamins, minerals, and omega-3 fatty acids, red snapper is as delicious as it is nutritious. Done my way, the fillets are coated with pistachios and paired with a sweet-and-salty maple-ginger glaze and baby carrots. You could easily enjoy the snapper on its own, although I also like to serve it over a bed of rice.

4 (4-ounce) red snapper fillets

¼ cup olive oil

3 tablespoons maple syrup

1 tablespoon balsamic vinegar

1 teaspoon minced ginger

1 teaspoon minced garlic

½ teaspoon paprika

Salt

Freshly ground black pepper

1 (1-pound) bag baby carrots

1 red onion, thinly sliced

½ lemon, thinly sliced, plus ½ lemon for juice

½ cup ground pistachios

1 teaspoon minced fresh parsley

1. Preheat the oven to 400°F.

2. Rinse the red snapper fillets with cold water, pat dry, and place onto a plate in the refrigerator until ready to cook.

3. In a small bowl, whisk together the olive oil, maple syrup, balsamic vinegar, ginger, garlic, and paprika. Season with salt and pepper.

4. Arrange the carrots on a sheet pan. Brush half the maple-ginger glaze over the carrots.

5. Bake for 15 minutes, then remove from the oven and toss the carrots using tongs.

6. Increase the oven temperature to 425°F.

7. Place the snapper fillets between the carrots on the sheet pan. Arrange the red onion and lemon slices around the carrots and the fillets.

8. Squeeze the juice from the other half of the lemon over the fish and carrots. Season with salt and pepper, then brush the rest of the glaze on top.

9. Bake in the oven for another 10 minutes, or until the fish flakes with a fork. Remove the pan from the oven, and rub the ground pistachios on top of the fish fillets, coating evenly.

10. Put the fish back in the oven and broil for 3 minutes, or until the pistachios are browned.

11. Garnish with fresh parsley, and serve.

Ingredient Tip: You can use regular carrots as well. Simply peel them, then slice into rounds.

Per Serving: Calories: 452; Saturated Fat: 3g; Total Fat: 23g; Protein: 35g; Total Carbs: 28g; Fiber: 6g; Sodium: 295mg

Roasted Cod and Sweet Potatoes

DAIRY-FREE, 5-INGREDIENT

SERVES 4 / PREP TIME: 15 MINUTES / COOK TIME: 45 MINUTES

Sometimes a simple combination of fresh ingredients prevails over a demanding preparation. This recipe is one such instance. Be sure to start cooking the potatoes first for a properly crispy texture. This dish may take a little while to put together, but after one bite, you'll realize it was worth the wait.

2 large sweet potatoes, peeled and thinly sliced

¼ cup olive oil, plus more for drizzling

4 garlic cloves, minced

1 teaspoon salt

1 teaspoon freshly ground black pepper

4 (6-ounce) cod fillets

1 lemon, thinly sliced

1. Preheat the oven to 425°F.
2. Line a sheet pan with parchment paper.
3. In a medium bowl, toss the sweet potatoes with the oil, garlic, salt, and pepper.
4. Place the sweet potatoes on the sheet pan in two even rows, to make a bed for the fish.
5. Bake for 30 minutes.
6. Remove from the oven, and place the cod fillets on top of the sweet potatoes. Drizzle with oil and top with lemon slices.
7. Bake for 15 minutes, or until the fish flakes with a fork. Serve warm.

Substitution Tip: You can use russet potatoes if you prefer them to sweet potatoes.

Per Serving: Calories: 305; Saturated Fat: 2g; Total Fat: 14g; Protein: 31g; Total Carbs: 14g; Fiber: 2g; Sodium: 732mg

Potato Chip-Crusted Salmon

DAIRY-FREE, 5-INGREDIENT, 30-MINUTE

SERVES 4 / PREP TIME: 10 MINUTES / COOK TIME: 15 MINUTES

Not only does using potato chips save time in the kitchen, it makes for a uniquely flavorful topping. This recipe ensures you'll cook the fish for just enough time, without burning the potato chips. Consider this dish a lighter, more creative, gluten-free twist on classic fish and chips.

4 (6-ounce) salmon fillets

1 (8.5-ounce) bag salt and vinegar potato chips

4 tablespoons Dijon mustard, divided

Salt

Freshly ground black pepper

1. Preheat the oven to 450°F.
2. Place the salmon fillets in a shallow 9-by-13-inch baking dish, lined with parchment paper.
3. Smash potato chips in a resealable bag.
4. Spread 1 tablespoon of the mustard over each fish fillet. Season with salt and pepper.
5. Top each fillet evenly with the crushed potato chips.
6. Bake for 15 minutes, or until the fish flakes with a fork. Serve and enjoy.

Ingredient Tip: The best salt and vinegar chips to use here are the Kettle Brand Sea Salt and Vinegar.

Per Serving: Calories: 609; Saturated Fat: 5g; Total Fat: 34g; Protein: 38g; Total Carbs: 31g; Fiber: 3g; Sodium: 653mg

Coconut-Coated Shrimp

DAIRY-FREE, 30-MINUTE

SERVES 4 / PREP TIME: 15 MINUTES / COOK TIME: 15 MINUTES

Dipping the shrimp in the egg whites makes the coconut mixture stick, producing a crispy exterior and juicy interior. Whip up the two-ingredient dipping sauce, and trust me—you will not be disappointed! If you're unfamiliar with spicy duck sauce, you're in for a treat (it can be found in the Asian section of the supermarket).

For the shrimp

2 cups sweetened shredded coconut

1½ cups gluten-free panko bread crumbs

1 cup liquid egg whites

1 teaspoon salt

1 teaspoon coarse ground pepper

1 teaspoon onion powder

1 pound peeled and deveined
  tail-on shrimp

Nonstick cooking spray

For the dipping sauce

½ cup spicy duck sauce

½ cup apricot preserves

To make the shrimp

1. Preheat the oven to 425°F.

2. Line a sheet pan with parchment paper.

3. In a shallow medium bowl, mix the coconut and bread crumbs.

4. In a medium bowl, mix together the egg whites, salt, pepper, and onion powder.

5. Dip each shrimp into the egg white mixture followed by the coconut mixture. Then place the shrimp on the sheet pan.

6. Spray the shrimp with nonstick cooking spray. Bake for 6 minutes, or until pink and opaque.

7. Flip each shrimp, spray with nonstick cooking spray, and bake another 6 minutes, or until golden brown. Serve with dipping sauce.

To make the dipping sauce

In a small bowl, combine the duck sauce and preserves, mixing well.

Per Serving: Calories: 528; Saturated Fat: 11g; Total Fat: 16g; Protein: 25g; Total Carbs: 73g; Fiber: 4g; Sodium: 1890mg

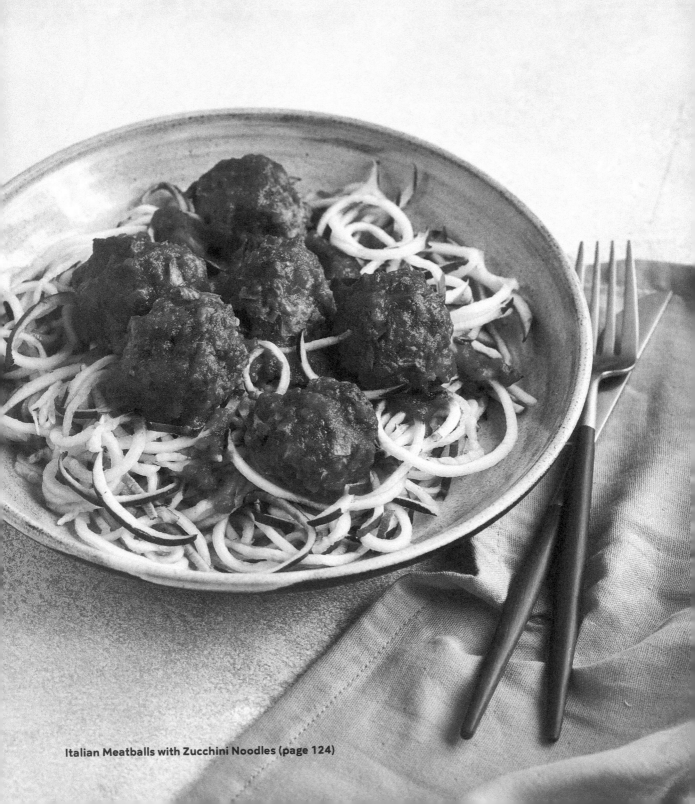

Italian Meatballs with Zucchini Noodles (page 124)

CHAPTER NINE

Poultry and Meat

Zesty Scallion Turkey Burgers

DAIRY-FREE

MAKES 6 BURGERS / PREP TIME: 10 MINUTES, PLUS 15 MINUTES TO CHILL / COOK TIME: 45 MINUTES

Many people hear turkey burger and think, "Oh, how boring." But these patties, spiced with sesame oil, scallions, and gluten-free soy sauce, are so delicious, they very well could change your opinion of turkey burgers for good. I recommend placing them on my Essential Sandwich Rolls (page 46) for the true burger experience.

3 tablespoons sesame oil, divided

1 cup cauliflower rice

4 scallions, chopped

2 garlic cloves, minced

1 tablespoon gluten-free soy sauce

2 pounds ground turkey

1 large egg

½ teaspoon onion powder

Dash salt

Pinch freshly ground black pepper

6 Essential Sandwich Rolls (optional)

1. In a medium skillet, heat 1 tablespoon of sesame oil over medium heat.

2. Add the cauliflower rice and sauté for 6 minutes. Add the scallions and garlic, and sauté for another 2 minutes, or until the garlic is fragrant. Stir in the soy sauce, then set aside to cool.

3. In a large bowl, combine the ground turkey, egg, onion powder, salt, and pepper.

4. Add the cauliflower mixture to the ground turkey and combine well. Using your hands, form the mixture into 6 patties.

5. Put the patties in the refrigerator for 15 minutes.

6. Heat the remaining 2 tablespoons of sesame oil in the skillet, and without overcrowding the pan, cook the burgers for 5 minutes per side over medium-high heat, or until browned. (If all 6 patties don't fit, cook them in batches.)

7. Cover the skillet and simmer the burgers over low heat for 10 minutes, or until the burgers are cooked through. Serve on Essential Sandwich Rolls (if using).

Make-Ahead Tip: I like to make these burgers in advance and freeze them for when I need a quick meal. Defrost them in the refrigerator in the morning before work, and they'll be ready to heat up for dinner by the time you get home.

Per Serving (1 burger): Calories: 248; Saturated Fat: 2g; Total Fat: 11g; Protein: 37g; Total Carbs: 2g; Fiber: 1g; Sodium: 277mg

Roasted Red Pepper Chicken

DAIRY-FREE, 5-INGREDIENT

SERVES 4 / PREP TIME: 15 MINUTES / COOK TIME: 1 HOUR 30 MINUTES, PLUS 5 MINUTES TO REST

This combination is so surprisingly delicious, I can hardly believe it was the result of a happy accident. I had set out to make tomato basil chicken, when I realized that what I had thrown in the food processor was a jar of roasted peppers instead of sundried tomatoes. To my surprise, the mixture had a much more intense flavor that paired incredibly well with the chicken.

1 (12-ounce) jar roasted red peppers

1 red bell pepper, seeded and quartered

1 cup Italian salad dressing

1 (1- to 2-pound) package bone-in chicken

1. Preheat the oven to 375°F.

2. In a food processor, combine the roasted red peppers, red bell pepper, and salad dressing. The ingredients should be combined, but the mixture should still be a bit chunky.

3. Place the chicken into a 9-by-13-inch baking dish.

4. Pour the pepper mixture over the chicken.

5. Bake for 1 hour 30 minutes, or until the chicken reaches an internal temperature of 165°F (or if you prefer more well done, 180°F).

6. Allow the chicken to rest for 5 minutes before serving.

Troubleshooting Tip: If you don't have a food processor, you can make the sauce in a blender.

Per Serving: Calories: 430; Saturated Fat: 4g; Total Fat: 23g; Protein: 43g; Total Carbs: 15g; Fiber: 1g; Sodium: 302mg

One-Pan Mediterranean Chicken and Veggies

DAIRY-FREE, 5-INGREDIENT

SERVES 4 / PREP TIME: 5 MINUTES / COOK TIME: 35 MINUTES, PLUS 5 MINUTES TO REST

I love sheet-pan meals, and once you see how easy they are to throw together, you will, too. Just throw a protein and some vegetables together on a pan, add some marinade, put it in the oven, and bam—you've got a delicious, healthy meal for the entire family.

2 pounds boneless chicken

2 tablespoons olive oil, divided

¼ cup Greek seasoning

2 heads cauliflower, chopped into florets

1 pint cherry tomatoes

2 sweet peppers, seeded and thinly sliced

½ teaspoon salt

¼ teaspoon freshly ground black pepper

Ingredient Tip: You can find Greek seasoning in the spice aisle of the grocery store, but if you'd prefer to make your own, mix together 1½ teaspoons of dried oregano, ½ teaspoon of dried basil, ½ teaspoon of dried marjoram, ¼ teaspoon of onion powder, and ¼ teaspoon of garlic powder.

Per Serving: Calories: 390; Saturated Fat: 1g; Total Fat: 11g; Protein: 57g; Total Carbs: 20g; Fiber: 5g; Sodium: 958mg

1. Preheat the oven to 425°F.

2. Put the chicken on a sheet pan, toss with 1 tablespoon of olive oil, then season with Greek seasoning.

3. Arrange the cauliflower, tomatoes, and peppers on the pan around the chicken. Sprinkle with salt and pepper, and drizzle with the remaining tablespoon of oil.

4. Roast for 30 minutes, or until the chicken reaches an internal temperature of 165°F (or if you prefer more well done, 180°F).

5. Remove the pan from the oven, cover with aluminum foil for 5 minutes, then serve.

Flank Steak "Noodle" Bowls

DAIRY-FREE

SERVES 2 / PREP TIME: 15 MINUTES / COOK TIME: 35 MINUTES

These noodle bowls share some flavors with a slightly sweet-and-salty Pad Thai, but unlike that classic dish, mine is packed with nutrition—particularly from the sweet potato and spinach, which provide a significant helping of antioxidants. Who knew eating steak could be so healthy?

¼ cup gluten-free soy sauce

2 tablespoons honey

1½ teaspoons sesame oil

1 pound flank steak, very thinly sliced

½ onion, very thinly sliced

4 tablespoons canola or vegetable oil, divided

1 large egg, beaten

2 scallions, green parts only, cut into 1-inch lengths

4 to 5 fresh mushrooms, very thinly sliced

6 ounces fresh baby spinach or baby kale

2 medium sweet potatoes, spiralized

1 tablespoon sesame seeds

1. In a small bowl, whisk together the soy sauce, honey, and sesame oil. Set aside.

2. In a large bowl, combine the flank steak and onion. Pour in about ⅓ of the soy sauce marinade. Set aside, allowing the beef and onions to marinate.

3. In a small skillet, heat 1 tablespoon of canola oil over medium heat. Add the beaten egg and scramble. Remove the skillet from the heat and set aside.

4. In a medium skillet, heat 1 tablespoon of canola oil over medium heat. Add the scallions, mushrooms, and baby spinach, and stir-fry for 5 minutes, or until tender. Transfer the vegetables to a separate bowl and set aside.

5. In the same skillet, heat 1 tablespoon of canola oil over medium heat. Sauté the sweet potatoes for 5 to 8 minutes, or until they become bright orange. Transfer the sweet potatoes to a separate bowl, and set aside.

6. In a large skillet, heat the remaining tablespoon of canola oil over medium-high heat. Add the marinated flank steak and onions, and cook for 6 to 8 minutes per side of the steak, or until the desired doneness is reached.

7. To assemble the bowls and serve, put all the ingredients into the large skillet and sauté for about 2 minutes, or until fully incorporated. Add the remaining marinade and sesame seeds to enjoy.

Troubleshooting Tip: A spiralizer is a great investment for your gluten-free kitchen. But if you don't have one, you can purchase pre-spiralized veggies in most supermarkets.

Per Serving: Calories: 964; Saturated Fat: 7g; Total Fat: 56g; Protein: 64g; Total Carbs: 56g; Fiber: 9g; Sodium: 2102mg

Roasted Olive Chicken

DAIRY-FREE

SERVES 4 / PREP TIME: 10 MINUTES / COOK TIME: 45 MINUTES, PLUS 5 MINUTES TO REST

This chicken dish more or less transforms your home kitchen into a fancy Greek restaurant. Roasting the chicken on the bone prevents the meat from drying out, and brings out the signature saltiness of the olives. Serve with garlic roasted potatoes for the total roasted chicken experience.

2 pounds bone-in chicken

1 (15-ounce) can pitted green olives, rinsed and drained

2 lemons, each cut into 8 slices

1 sweet onion, chopped

3 tablespoons olive oil

1 teaspoon paprika

½ teaspoon garlic powder

½ teaspoon salt

¼ teaspoon freshly ground black pepper

1. Preheat the oven to 400°F.

2. Arrange the chicken, olives, lemon slices, and onion on a sheet pan.

3. In a small bowl, mix the oil with the paprika, garlic powder, salt, and pepper.

4. Evenly coat the chicken, olives, lemon slices, and onion with the oil mixture.

5. Roast for 45 minutes, or until the chicken reaches an internal temperature of 165°F (or if you prefer more well done, 180°F).

6. Allow the chicken to rest for 5 minutes, then serve.

Make-Ahead Tip: You can prepare this recipe in the morning before you leave for work and pop it in the oven when you return. In the morning, just follow steps 2 through 4, cover the sheet pan with aluminum foil, then refrigerate. When you get home, preheat the oven to 400°F, take out the sheet pan, uncover, and roast.

Per Serving: Calories: 561; Saturated Fat: 9g; Total Fat: 40g; Protein: 45g; Total Carbs: 7g; Fiber: 3g; Sodium: 1059mg

Crispy Fried Chicken Cutlets

DAIRY-FREE, 30-MINUTE

SERVES 4 / PREP TIME: 20 MINUTES / COOK TIME: 10 MINUTES

Nobody can turn down fried chicken—and that includes this gluten-free version. Chickpea flour helps create a crisp texture, although coconut flour works as well. I like to make fried cutlets, so they can be repurposed in a variety of ways. They're great chopped up over salad, in a sandwich, or laid on top of rice.

2 pounds chicken cutlets

Salt

Freshly ground black pepper

2 large eggs

1 teaspoon gluten-free soy sauce

1 teaspoon Sriracha (or hot sauce of your choice)

1 cup chickpea flour

½ cup potato starch

1 teaspoon onion powder

1 teaspoon garlic powder

1 teaspoon paprika

½ teaspoon dried parsley

2 tablespoons flavor-neutral oil

1. Season the chicken with salt and pepper.

2. In a small bowl, mix together the eggs, soy sauce, and Sriracha.

3. In a medium bowl, mix together the flour, potato starch, onion powder, garlic powder, paprika, and parsley.

4. Line a large plate (or a sheet pan works nicely) with paper towels, and a second large plate with parchment paper.

5. Coat each chicken cutlet first in the egg mixture followed by the flour mixture. Place each cutlet on the parchment-covered plate, repeating until all of the cutlets are coated.

6. Heat the oil in a large skillet over medium heat. Without overcrowding the pan, fry the cutlets for about 4 minutes per side, or until golden brown and cooked through. (If all the cutlets don't fit in the skillet, cook them in batches.) Place the finished cutlets on the paper towel-lined plate to absorb the excess oil, then serve.

Ingredient Tip: If you like your fried chicken a little sweeter, you can drizzle with honey and reheat quickly, so the honey melts.

Per Serving: Calories: 501; Saturated Fat: 2g; Total Fat: 14g; Protein: 61g; Total Carbs: 32g; Fiber: 5g; Sodium: 274mg

Honey Teriyaki Chicken Wings

DAIRY-FREE, 5-INGREDIENT

SERVES 4 / PREP TIME: 10 MINUTES / COOK TIME: 25 MINUTES

Unlike traditional chicken wings, these are baked rather than fried, making them healthier (in addition to being gluten-free). Combining teriyaki sauce with honey produces a sweet and salty flavor, while contributing to the signature stickiness that makes wings so much fun to eat. They're so insanely addictive, you might want to go ahead and double the recipe.

For the honey teriyaki sauce

1 (10-ounce) bottle teriyaki sauce

¾ cup honey

For the chicken wings

3 pounds chicken wings (about 15)

4 scallions, chopped

2 tablespoons sesame seeds

> **Make-Ahead Tip:** You can clean the wings, marinate them in the sauce, and refrigerate them up to 24 hours before baking. You can also refrigerate any extra sauce for up to one week.

Per Serving: Calories: 882; Saturated Fat: 11g; Total Fat: 42g; Protein: 42g; Total Carbs: 86g; Fiber: 2g; Sodium: 3310mg

To make the honey teriyaki sauce

In a medium bowl, combine the teriyaki sauce and honey, stirring well.

To make the chicken wings

1. Preheat the oven to 450°F.
2. Line two sheet pans with parchment paper.
3. Pour half of the honey teriyaki sauce into a large bowl. Toss the wings in the sauce, coating them thoroughly.
4. Place the wings on the sheet pans and bake for 15 minutes.
5. Flip the wings, drizzle with more sauce, then return to the oven for another 10 minutes.
6. Top with chopped scallions and sesame seeds, and serve with the remaining sauce on the side.

Shirataki Noodles with Turkey Sausage

DAIRY-FREE, 30-MINUTE

SERVES 4 / PREP TIME: 10 MINUTES / COOK TIME: 20 MINUTES

Shirataki noodles are one of the most underestimated ingredients for a gluten-free kitchen. They are naturally gluten-free, low in calories, and super easy and quick to prepare. Their mild flavor makes them an ideal base for any tasty protein, but I love to pair them with turkey sausage. You'll find them in the refrigerated section of the produce aisle in the supermarket, typically near the tofu.

1 (7-ounce) package shirataki noodles

2 pounds ground turkey sausage

¼ cup balsamic vinegar

3 tablespoons Dijon mustard

Dash salt

Pinch freshly ground black pepper

9 ounces fresh baby spinach

½ cup chopped walnuts

1 pear, thinly sliced

Ingredient Tip: Shirataki noodles are made from a Japanese plant called konjac. These noodles are very low in calories, although they do contain fiber. They can be rinsed and dried, then put directly into a sauce. However, they tend to taste better if they are dried over heat in a skillet first.

Per Serving: Calories: 425; Saturated Fat: 1g; Total Fat: 24g; Protein: 37g; Total Carbs: 16g; Fiber: 5g; Sodium: 1336mg

1. Drain the shirataki noodles, then rinse with hot water and drain again.

2. In a medium skillet, cook the noodles over medium-low heat for about 6 minutes, or until they are dry. Once done, distribute the noodles evenly among 4 serving bowls.

3. In the same skillet, sauté the sausage over medium-high heat for about 10 minutes, or until brown and cooked through.

4. In a small bowl, whisk together the vinegar, mustard, salt, and pepper.

5. Top each bowl of noodles with the spinach, walnuts, and pears. Finally, add the sausage.

6. Drizzle the dressing on top, and serve.

Sticky Glazed Pork Chops and Spinach

DAIRY-FREE, 5-INGREDIENT

SERVES 4 / PREP TIME: 10 MINUTES / COOK TIME: 25 MINUTES

The combination of soda and hoisin in this recipe works together to create a sweet, tangy flavor. If you want to expand on the Caribbean-inspired sweetness, adding coconut rice would work very well. Just replace the water with coconut milk when you're making the rice.

4 thinly cut pork chops

Salt

Freshly ground black pepper

4 tablespoons flavor-neutral oil, divided

7 ounces fresh baby spinach

1 can Dr. Pepper soda

⅔ cup gluten-free hoisin sauce

2 tablespoons water

1. Season the pork chops with salt and pepper. Using a fork, poke some holes in the fat of the pork.

2. In a large skillet, heat 2 tablespoons of oil over medium heat. Sauté the spinach for 3 to 4 minutes, or until wilted. Season with salt and pepper, then transfer the spinach to a large bowl.

3. Add the remaining 2 tablespoons of oil to the skillet and sauté the pork chops for 5 minutes per side, or until browned and cooked through. Transfer the pork chops to a plate, and set aside.

4. Add the soda, hoisin, and water to the skillet and bring to a boil. Reduce the heat and simmer for about 3 minutes, until thickened.

5. Return the pork chops to the skillet and cook for 2 minutes, until coated with the sauce. Serve over the wilted spinach.

Substitution Tip: If you do not like pork, you can substitute veal chops or lamb shoulder chops.

Per Serving: Calories: 501; Saturated Fat: 6g; Total Fat: 29g; Protein: 27g; Total Carbs: 34g; Fiber: 1g; Sodium: 1504mg

Rosemary-Crusted Lamb

DAIRY-FREE, 5-INGREDIENT

SERVES 4 / PREP TIME: 5 MINUTES / COOK TIME: 1 HOUR 30 MINUTES, PLUS 5 MINUTES TO REST

This absolutely stunning lamb dish is sure to be a crowd pleaser. Racks of lamb are such a delicious cut of meat; all they really require is a simple seasoning to bring out their natural flavors. If you'd prefer to work with lamb chops, you can season them the same way and broil on a sheet pan for 5 minutes on each side.

6-pound rack of lamb

¼ cup olive oil

6 garlic cloves, minced

1½ teaspoons dried rosemary

1 teaspoon salt

1 teaspoon freshly ground black pepper

1. Preheat the oven to 325°F.

2. Place the lamb in a 9-by-13-inch baking dish.

3. In a small bowl, mix together the olive oil, garlic, rosemary, salt, and pepper.

4. Rub the oil mixture over the lamb.

5. Bake for 15 minutes per pound, or 1 hour 30 minutes total for medium rare.

6. Allow the lamb to rest for 5 minutes before serving.

Troubleshooting Tip: If you prefer your lamb well-done, bake for up to 30 minutes per pound (or 3 hours). But most people enjoy lamb medium rare to medium, which would require roasting for no longer than 20 minutes per pound.

Per Serving: Calories: 837; Saturated Fat: 15g; Total Fat: 48g; Protein: 92g; Total Carbs: 1g; Fiber: 0g; Sodium: 708mg

Italian Meatballs with Zucchini Noodles

DAIRY-FREE

SERVES 4 / PREP TIME: 10 MINUTES / COOK TIME: 1 HOUR 20 MINUTES

I like to make the meatballs in the sauce, a technique that flavors the sauce and reduces the fat necessary for panfrying. Serve this dish with a simple green salad and red wine, and you've got yourself a perfect Italian dinner.

2 tablespoons olive oil

½ (10-ounce) bag frozen riced mixed vegetables

2 pounds ground beef

2 large eggs

½ teaspoon salt

¼ teaspoon freshly ground black pepper

2 (16-ounce) jars marinara sauce

4 garlic cloves, minced

4 zucchini, spiralized

1. In a medium skillet, heat the oil over medium heat. Add the riced vegetables, and sauté for about 8 minutes, or until warmed and golden brown. Set aside to cool.

2. In a large bowl, combine the ground beef, eggs, salt, and pepper.

3. Pour the marinara sauce into a large saucepan, then add the minced garlic. Cover and bring the sauce to a boil over high heat.

4. Combine the riced vegetables and ground beef mixture. Using your hands, form 24 meatballs about 1 inch in diameter.

5. Put the meatballs in the boiling sauce, cover, and simmer on low heat for 1 hour, or until the meatballs are cooked through.

6. Put the zucchini spirals in a large microwave-safe bowl. Microwave the zucchini noodles for 3 minutes, then spoon evenly into 4 bowls.

7. Top the noodles with the meatballs and sauce, then serve.

Substitution Tip: You can always substitute sprialized carrots, sweet potatoes, beets, or parsnips.

Per Serving: Calories: 531; Saturated Fat: 8g; Total Fat: 26g; Protein: 53g; Total Carbs: 26g; Fiber: 7g; Sodium: 1804mg

Beef Tenderloin and Crispy Kale

DAIRY-FREE, 5-INGREDIENT, 30-MINUTE

SERVES 4 / PREP TIME: 15 MINUTES / COOK TIME: 6 MINUTES, PLUS 5 MINUTES TO REST

This quick and easy recipe makes a great weeknight dinner—but who says weeknights have to be boring? The combination of mouth-watering tenderloin with the sweet beets and crisp kale is wonderful. Plus, this dish makes a dramatically colorful and elegant presentation—so elegant, in fact, that you might consider saving it for your next dinner party.

1 bunch beets, peeled and thinly sliced

1 bunch kale, stemmed and torn into bite-size pieces

3½ tablespoons olive oil

4 (8-to-10-ounce) beef tenderloin filets

¼ teaspoon Italian seasoning

Pinch salt

Dash freshly ground black pepper

1. Preheat the broiler on low heat.

2. In a large bowl, toss the beets and kale with the olive oil to coat.

3. Place the vegetables and filets together on a sheet pan, and season both with Italian seasoning, salt, and pepper.

4. Put the sheet pan in the oven and broil for 2 to 3 minutes.

5. Remove the sheet pan from the oven. Flip each filet over and broil for another 2 to 3 minutes, or until the filets are cooked medium rare, the beets are tender, and the kale is crisp.

6. Remove the sheet pan from the oven, and allow the beef to rest for 5 minutes before serving.

Ingredient Tip: To save time, you can buy precooked and peeled beets, which are available in most supermarkets.

Per Serving: Calories: 549; Saturated Fat: 7g; Total Fat: 27g; Protein: 55g; Total Carbs: 22g; Fiber: 4g; Sodium: 311mg

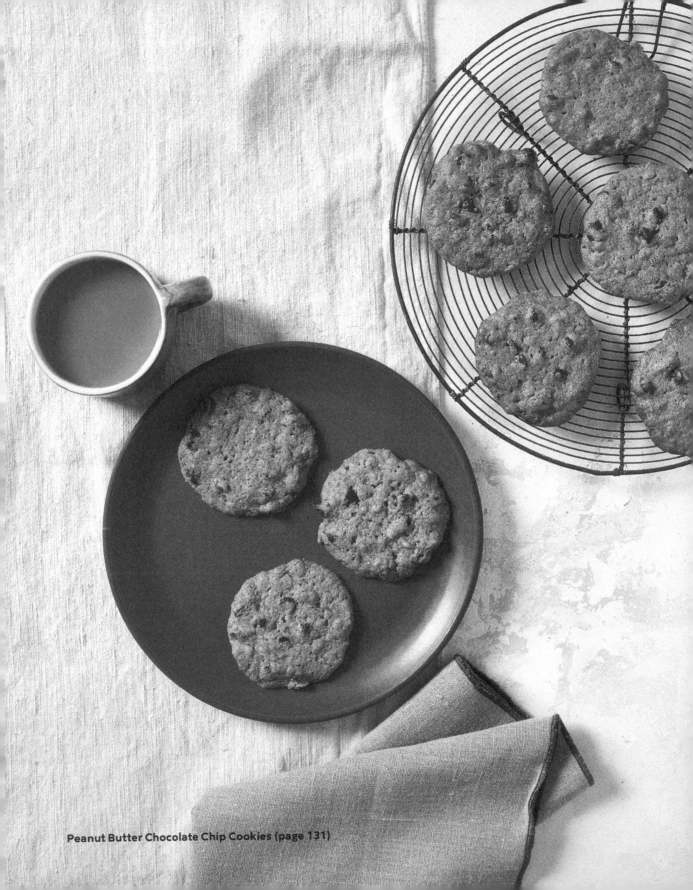

Peanut Butter Chocolate Chip Cookies (page 131)

CHAPTER TEN
Desserts

Coconut Rice Pudding

VEGETARIAN, 5-INGREDIENT

SERVES 4 / PREP TIME: 20 MINUTES / COOK TIME: 1 HOUR, PLUS 30 MINUTES TO COOL

This recipe updates the classic with the addition of coconut milk. If you're making a rice dish for dinner, make a little extra rice and use it for this delicious dessert.

¾ cup uncooked rice

1½ cups water

1 (14-ounce) can full-fat coconut milk

1½ cups whole milk

½ cup sugar

Pinch salt

½ teaspoon vanilla extract

Substitution Tip: To make this dairy-free, substitute the whole milk with a non-dairy alternative, such as almond milk.

Per Serving: Calories: 507; Saturated Fat: 23g; Total Fat: 27g; Protein: 8g; Total Carbs: 63g; Fiber: 3g; Sodium: 92mg

1. Add the rice to a small bowl and rinse with water. Drain the rice through a fine mesh strainer, and transfer to a medium saucepan.

2. Add the water to the saucepan and bring to a boil over high heat.

3. Turn the heat to medium-high and cook until most of the water is absorbed, about 5 minutes. Cover the pan, turn the heat to low, and simmer for 10 minutes, or until the rest of the water is absorbed. Remove from the heat, uncover, and cool for 30 minutes. The cooked rice should yield 1½ cups.

4. In a medium pot, combine the cooked rice, coconut milk, whole milk, sugar, and salt.

5. Simmer over medium heat, stirring frequently, until thickened (about 40 minutes).

6. Mix in the vanilla and serve.

Very Blueberry Pie

VEGETARIAN

SERVES 4, WITH LEFTOVERS / PREP TIME: 15 MINUTES / COOK TIME: 45 MINUTES

I'll always be partial to blueberry pie, because it brings back childhood memories of picking wild blueberries in Maine. But this pie recipe will work well with really any fruit, from peaches to apples to pears.

2 pints blueberries

1 Essential Pie Crust (page 48)

2 cups sugar, divided

2 cups gluten-free oats

1 cup almond flour

¾ cup coconut oil, at room temperature

4 tablespoons unsalted butter, at room temperature

2 teaspoons ground cinnamon

1. Preheat the oven to 350°F.

2. Pat the blueberries with paper towel to dry up any moisture, then spread them evenly over the pie crust. Sprinkle with ½ cup sugar.

3. In a medium bowl, mix together the remaining 1½ cups sugar, the oats, almond flour, coconut oil, butter, and cinnamon.

4. Sprinkle the crumb topping mixture on top of the berries.

5. Bake for 45 minutes, or until the fruit is bubbling. Serve and enjoy.

Make-Ahead Tip: Prepare the crust and topping ahead of time, and keep them in the freezer for whenever you want to make a pie at a moment's notice.

Per Serving: Calories: 1275; Saturated Fat: 49g; Total Fat: 77g; Protein: 12g; Total Carbs: 148g; Fiber: 10g; Sodium: 299mg

Meringue Cookies

DAIRY-FREE, VEGETARIAN, 5-INGREDIENT

MAKES 12 COOKIES / PREP TIME: 15 MINUTES / COOK TIME: 25 MINUTES

Meringues are naturally gluten-free, with a texture that starts out crunchy, turns a bit chewy, then melts in your mouth. All you need are egg whites and a few other ingredients to whip up these cookies. And if you have any left over, you can crumble them up and use them as a topping for the Chocolate Mousse (page 133).

2 egg whites

½ teaspoon cream of tartar

Pinch salt

½ cup sugar

1 teaspoon white vinegar

½ teaspoon vanilla extract

Ingredient Tip: To separate egg whites from yolks, crack each egg one at a time and carefully move the yolk back and forth between the two halves of the shell, letting the white of the egg drip into a bowl below.

Per Serving (2 cookies): Calories: 70; Saturated Fat: 0g; Total Fat: 0g; Protein: 2g; Total Carbs: 18g; Fiber: 0g; Sodium: 34mg

1. Preheat the oven to 225°F.
2. Line a sheet pan with parchment paper.
3. Crack the eggs, and separate the whites into a medium bowl.
4. Using a hand mixer, beat the egg whites with the cream of tartar and salt, until soft peaks form and they stand up when the mixer is lifted.
5. Add the sugar slowly, continuing to beat until stiff peaks form.
6. Fold in the vinegar and vanilla.
7. Place teaspoon-size dollops of the mixture on the prepared pan.
8. Bake for 25 minutes.
9. Turn off the oven, and let the meringues cool in the oven before serving.

Peanut Butter Chocolate Chip Cookies

DAIRY-FREE, VEGETARIAN, 30-MINUTE

MAKES 12 TO 15 COOKIES / PREP TIME: 10 MINUTES / COOK TIME: 15 MINUTES

You don't have to give up favorites like peanut butter chocolate chip cookies, just because you can't eat gluten. I recommend making a great big batch and keeping them in the freezer. They'll stay fresh there for a few months, but I'd be shocked if they weren't eaten up long before that. One of my favorite ways to use these cookies is as buns for an ice cream sandwich. Just stuff your favorite flavor between two, and you're good to go!

1 cup sugar

1 cup peanut butter

1 cup semisweet chocolate chips

⅓ cup gluten-free oats

¼ cup vegetable oil

2 large eggs

1 teaspoon vanilla extract

½ teaspoon baking powder

Pinch salt

1. Preheat the oven to 325°F.

2. Line a sheet pan with parchment paper.

3. In a large bowl, mix together the sugar, peanut butter, chocolate chips, oats, oil, eggs, vanilla, baking powder, and salt.

4. Using a tablespoon, drop the cookie dough onto the sheet pan.

5. Bake for about 15 minutes, or until just golden brown. Cool before serving.

Substitution Tip: If you're concerned about peanut allergies, you can substitute almond butter or any other nut butter for the peanut butter.

Per Serving (2 cookies): Calories: 684; Saturated Fat: 12g; Total Fat: 41g; Protein: 16g; Total Carbs: 70g; Fiber: 12g; Sodium: 268mg

Pecan Squares

VEGETARIAN

MAKES 12 SQUARES / PREP TIME: 10 MINUTES / COOK TIME: 55 MINUTES

"Pecan squares." For me, just saying those two words conjures up memories of the holiday season. These treats are surprisingly easy to make—and they're so good, I guarantee nobody will notice they're gluten-free.

Nonstick cooking spray

1¼ cups Jamie's Whole-Grain Flour Blend (page 45)

⅓ cup sugar, plus ½ cup

2⅓ cups chopped pecans, divided

8 tablespoons (1 stick) unsalted butter, at room temperature, divided

⅓ cup corn syrup

1 large egg

2 tablespoons water

2 teaspoons vanilla extract

Pinch salt

1. Preheat the oven to 350°F.

2. Spray a 9-by-9-inch baking dish with nonstick cooking spray, and line with parchment paper.

3. To prepare the crust, combine the flour blend, ⅓ cup of sugar, and ⅓ cup of pecans in a food processor until well mixed.

4. Put 4 tablespoons of butter in the food processor, and mix until the dough becomes the consistency of wet sand.

5. Press the dough into the prepared pan. Bake for 25 minutes, or until golden brown. Set aside to cool.

6. Melt the remaining 4 tablespoons of butter in the microwave.

7. To prepare the filling, in a large bowl, combine the melted butter, ½ cup of sugar, corn syrup, egg, water, vanilla extract, and salt.

8. Pour the filling over the cooled crust. Top with the remaining 2 cups of pecans.

9. Bake for 30 minutes, or until the filling is set. Cut into 12 equal-size squares before serving.

Substitution Tip: For a simple variation, try the recipe with walnuts instead of pecans.

Per Serving (1 square): Calories: 373; Saturated Fat: 7g; Total Fat: 23g; Protein: 4g; Total Carbs: 41g; Fiber: 2g; Sodium: 73mg

Chocolate Mousse

DAIRY-FREE, VEGETARIAN, 5-INGREDIENT, 30-MINUTE

SERVES 2 / PREP TIME: 10 MINUTES, PLUS OVERNIGHT TO SEPARATE CREAM

Leading a healthy lifestyle doesn't mean eliminating chocolate. This mousse is naturally gluten-free, surprisingly light, and absolutely delicious. It couldn't be easier to make, and it's always a crowd-pleaser. You can keep it in the refrigerator for a few days after you make it to satisfy late-night chocolate cravings. To get extra fancy, try serving it in a martini glass, garnished with raspberries.

1 (14-ounce) can full-fat coconut milk, chilled in the refrigerator overnight

3 tablespoons cocoa powder

2 tablespoons maple syrup

Raspberries, for garnish

1. The night before making the mousse, refrigerate the can of coconut milk overnight so the cream and liquid separate.

2. Scoop the cream into a blender. Discard the liquid.

3. Blend the cream with the cocoa powder and maple syrup until completely smooth.

4. Store in the refrigerator for 3 to 4 days, or serve right away with raspberries.

Make-Ahead Tip: Because you can store this mousse in a covered bowl in the refrigerator and enjoy it over several days, you might want to double the recipe.

Per Serving: Calories: 284; Saturated Fat: 10g; Total Fat: 11g; Protein: 2g; Total Carbs: 50g; Fiber: 3g; Sodium: 25mg

Dark Chocolate Bark with Pumpkin and Pecans

DAIRY-FREE, VEGETARIAN, 5-INGREDIENT, 30-MINUTE

SERVES 8 / PREP TIME: 10 MINUTES / COOK TIME: 10 MINUTES, PLUS 30 MINUTES TO HARDEN

This recipe is one you'll probably want to double, so you can store some chocolate bark in the freezer. Just be forewarned: It will be difficult to keep yourself from sneaking bites throughout the day. I recommend using pumpkin seeds and pecans, but feel free to change up the toppings with different dried fruits, coconut, and nuts.

1 (10-ounce) package dark chocolate chips

½ cup pumpkin seeds

½ cup chopped pecans

1. Line a sheet pan with parchment paper.

2. In a large saucepan, heat about 2 inches (or 1 cup) of water on high heat, until boiling.

3. Place a small saucepan inside the large saucepan. Put the chocolate in the smaller saucepan.

4. Stirring constantly, heat the chocolate on medium heat for about 4 minutes, or until the chocolate melts.

5. Immediately spread the melted chocolate over the parchment-lined pan.

6. Sprinkle with pumpkin seeds and pecans.

7. Put the pan in the freezer or set aside and allow it to harden for 30 minutes. Break into cookie-size pieces, and store what you don't serve in a resealable bag in the refrigerator.

Troubleshooting Tip: In step 3, you're effectively using a double-boil method, which is a great way to melt chocolate so it doesn't burn. If you happen to have a double boiler, feel free to use it instead.

Per Serving: Calories: 257; Saturated Fat: 7g; Total Fat: 18g; Protein: 5g; Total Carbs: 26g; Fiber: 1g; Sodium: 2mg

Super Gooey Chocolate Brownies

DAIRY-FREE, VEGETARIAN

MAKES 8 BROWNIES / PREP: 15 MINUTES / COOK: 35 MINUTES

It's become a trend to bake desserts with vegetable alternatives, and for good reason: Not only are they delicious, but they offer a healthier way to indulge. These brownies are made with zucchini. You won't taste it at all, but it will contribute to the terrifically moist texture of the brownies.

Nonstick cooking spray

1 cup shredded zucchini

1 (12-ounce) package chocolate chips

½ cup flavor-neutral oil

1 teaspoon vanilla extract

½ cup applesauce

3 large eggs

1½ cups sugar

1 cup Jamie's All-Purpose Flour Blend (page 44)

1 teaspoon baking powder

1 teaspoon xanthan gum

¼ teaspoon salt

½ cup chopped walnuts

Troubleshooting Tip: If you do not have a food processor to shred the zucchini, you can buy spiralized zucchini in the supermarket and finely chop it.

Per Serving (1 brownie): Calories: 618; Saturated Fat: 12g; Total Fat: 35g; Protein: 8g; Total Carbs: 65g; Fiber: 4g; Sodium: 103mg

1. Preheat the oven to 350°F.

2. Line an 8-by-8-inch baking dish with parchment paper, and coat with nonstick cooking spray.

3. In a large bowl, add the shredded zucchini, making sure it's squeezed of all excess moisture.

4. In a large, microwave-safe bowl, microwave the chocolate chips, oil, and vanilla for 2 minutes on medium heat, or until the chocolate chips are completely melted. Remove the bowl from the microwave.

5. Add the zucchini, applesauce, and eggs to the chocolate mixture, and mix well.

6. Mix in the sugar, flour blend, baking powder, xanthan gum, and salt, stirring until well blended. Fold in the walnuts.

7. Pour the batter into the prepared pan.

8. Bake for 30 to 35 minutes, or until a toothpick inserted into the center comes out with just a few crumbs attached (it should not be completely wet, but a little gooeyness is fine).

9. Allow the brownies to cool completely. Cut them into 8 equal-size rectangles before serving.

MEASUREMENTS AND CONVERSIONS

VOLUME EQUIVALENTS (LIQUID)

US STANDARD	US STANDARD (OUNCES)	METRIC (APPROXIMATE)
2 tablespoons	1 fl. oz.	30 mL
¼ cup	2 fl. oz.	60 mL
½ cup	4 fl. oz.	120 mL
1 cup	8 fl. oz.	240 mL
1½ cups	12 fl. oz.	355 mL
2 cups or 1 pint	16 fl. oz.	475 mL
4 cups or 1 quart	32 fl. oz.	1 L
1 gallon	128 fl. oz.	4 L

OVEN TEMPERATURES

FAHRENHEIT	CELSIUS (APPROXIMATE)
250°F	120°C
300°F	150°C
325°F	165°C
350°F	180°C
375°F	190°C
400°F	200°C
425°F	220°C
450°F	230°C

VOLUME EQUIVALENTS (DRY)

US STANDARD	METRIC (APPROXIMATE)
⅛ teaspoon	0.5 mL
¼ teaspoon	1 mL
½ teaspoon	2 mL
¾ teaspoon	4 mL
1 teaspoon	5 mL
1 tablespoon	15 mL
¼ cup	59 mL
⅓ cup	79 mL
½ cup	118 mL
⅔ cup	156 mL
¾ cup	177 mL
1 cup	235 mL
2 cups or 1 pint	475 mL
3 cups	700 mL
4 cups or 1 quart	1 L

WEIGHT EQUIVALENTS

US STANDARD	METRIC (APPROXIMATE)
½ ounce	15 g
1 ounce	30 g
2 ounces	60 g
4 ounces	115 g
8 ounces	225 g
12 ounces	340 g
16 ounces or 1 pound	455 g

MASTER LIST OF SAFE/UNSAFE INGREDIENTS

This list was adapted from three sources: Celiac.com, the Celiac Disease Foundation, and the Gluten Free Society.

SAFE INGREDIENTS

For Baking
- Guar gum
- Xanthan gum

Grains
- Amaranth*
- Buckwheat*
- Chia
- Flaxseed
- Hominy
- Millet
- Quinoa*
- Rice
- Sorghum*

Flours
- Almond
- Arrowroot
- Banana
- Buckwheat*
- Chickpea
- Coconut
- Corn*
- Millet*
- Gluten-free oats*
- Potato
- Quinoa*
- Rice
- Sorghum*
- Tapioca
- Teff*

Fresh, non-processed foods
- Beans
- Dairy (milk, cheese, yogurt, with nothing added), excluding blue cheeses
- Eggs
- Fish
- Fruits
- Meat
- Poultry
- Vegetables (including all starchy vegetables, such as corn, peas, potatoes, and squash)
- Wine

*Indicates ingredients that are naturally gluten-free, yet must feature gluten-free label on packaging, due to potential cross-contamination in the fields where they are grown or factories where they are processed.

UNSAFE INGREDIENTS

Barley

- Barley extract
- Barley grass
- Barley malt
- Malted barley flour
- Pearl barley
- Sprouted barley

Bran

Brewer's yeast

Bulgur

Caramel coloring (outside of the United States)

Cereal germ

Couscous

Edible coatings

Edible films

Hing (or heeng)

Kecap (or ketjap) manis (sweet soy sauce)

Malt

- Malted alcoholic beverages
- Malted milk
- Malt extract
- Malt flavoring
- Malt syrup
- Malt vinegar

Rice malt (or brown rice syrup)

Rye

Vegetable gum

Wheat

- Atta flour
- Bleached flour
- Bread flour
- Brown flour
- Bulgur wheat
- Club wheat
- Common wheat (also known as *Triticum aestivum* or *Triticum vulgare*)
- Durum (also known as pasta wheat or macaroni wheat)
- Edible starch flour
- Einkorn
- Emmer
- Emulsifying wheat proteins
- Enriched flour
- Farro
- Farina
- Frikeh (also known as, farik, fereek, or freekeh)
- Fu (Japanese dried wheat gluten)
- Graham flour
- Granary flour
- Groats
- Hard wheat
- Hydrolyzed wheat proteins
- Kamut
- Macha wheat
- Maida
- Matzo (or matza)
- Modified food starch (made from wheat)
- Oriental wheat
- Persian wheat
- Polish wheat
- Poulard wheat
- Rusk
- Self-rising flour
- Semolina
- Shot wheat
- Spelt
- Sprouted wheat
- Strong flour
- Timopheevii wheat
- Triticale
- Unbleached flour
- Vavilovi wheat
- Vital wheat gluten
- Wheat amino acids
- Wheat bran extract
- Wheat bulgur
- Wheat durum triticum
- Wheat germ (extracts, glycerides, oils)
- Wheat grass
- Wheat nuts
- Wheat protein
- Wheat starch
- Whole meal flour
- Wild einkorn
- Wild emmer

All of the following products and ingredients *can* be gluten-free, but must have, or be listed on a product that has, a gluten-free label in order to be safe to consume:

- Artificial color and flavor
- Baking powder
- Barbecue sauce
- Beer
- Blue cheese
- Bouillon cubes
- Bread
- Bread crumbs
- Brewer's yeast
- Brown rice syrup
- Bulgur
- Cakes
- Candy
- Cereal
- Cheese spreads
- Chocolate
- Clarifying agents
- Coloring
- Communion wafers
- Cookie crumbs
- Cookie dough
- Cookie dough pieces
- Cookies
- Crackers
- Crisped rice
- Croutons
- Deli meats (processed or pre-seasoned)
- Dip mixes
- Dry roasted nuts
- Dumplings
- Egg substitutes
- Emulsifiers
- Fat replacers
- Flavored chips
- Flour tortillas
- Food stabilizers
- French fries
- Granola bars
- Gravy cubes
- Ground spices
- Honey ham
- Honey roasted nuts
- Hot dogs
- Ice cream
- Imitation meats and fish
- Instant coffee
- Malt products
- Matzoh (or matza)
- Miso
- Modified food starch (if not made from wheat)
- Multigrain chips
- Multigrain rice cakes
- Mustard powder
- Non-dairy creamer
- Oats
- Panko bread crumbs
- Pasta
- Pizza
- Powder mixes
- Pregelatinized starch
- Pretzels
- Processed cheeses
- Puddings
- Ramen noodles
- Salad dressings
- Seafood analogs
- Seasonings (spices, herbs, and smoke flavoring)
- Seitan
- Self-basting meat
- Snack foods
- Soba noodles
- Soups, store-bought
- Sour cream
- Soy sauce
- Soy sauce solids
- Starch
- Stilton cheese
- Stock cubes
- Suet
- Surimi
- Teas
- Teriyaki sauce
- Tocopherols
- Vegetable broth
- Vegetable protein
- Vegetable starch
- Worcestershire sauce

The labels of these non-food items must be checked to make sure they do not contain gluten (or any gluten-containing ingredients):

Detergent

Envelopes

Hairspray

Herbal supplements

Lipstick, lip gloss, and lip balm

Makeup

Medications (prescription and over-the-counter)

Mouthwash

Nutrition supplements

Pet food

Playdough

Shampoo

Stamps

Toothpaste

RESOURCES

Books

Gluten Free: The Definitive Resource Guide by Shelley Case

A variety of gluten-free cookbooks by Nicole Hunn

2019 Gluten-Free Buyer's Guide by Josh Schieffer

Magazines

GFF Magazine: https://gffmag.com

Gluten-Free Living: https://www.glutenfreeliving.com

Websites

Beyond Celiac: https://www.beyondceliac.org

Celiac Disease Center at Columbia University Medical Center:
    Phone # 212-305-5590 / https://celiacdiseasecenter.columbia.edu

Celiac Disease Foundation: https://celiac.org

Celiac Society: http://www.celiacsociety.com

Gluten Free & More: https://www.glutenfreeandmore.com

Gluten Free Passport: https://glutenfreepassport.com

Gluten Free Travel Blog: https://glutenfreetravelblog.typepad.com

Gluten Intolerance Group: https://gluten.org

National Celiac Association: https://nationalceliac.org

National Institute of Diabetes and Digestive and Kidney Diseases:
    https://www.celiac.nih.gov

The University of Chicago Celiac Disease Center: Phone # 773-702-7593 /
    https://www.cureceliacdisease.org

Thrive Market: https://thrivemarket.com, Online market membership that delivers
    and has great prices, as well as a terrific variety of gluten-free products

REFERENCES

Adams, Scott. "Unsafe Gluten-Free Food List (Unsafe Ingredients)." Celiac.com, August 8, 2018. https://www.celiac.com/articles.html/unsafe-gluten-free-food-list -unsafe-ingredients-r182/.

Celiac Disease Foundation. "Sources of Gluten." Accessed November 21, 2019. https://celiac.org/gluten-free-living/what-is-gluten/sources-of-gluten/.

Gluten Free Society. "Guidelines for Avoiding Gluten (Unsafe Ingredients for Gluten Sensitivity)." March 20, 2018. https://www.glutenfreesociety.org/guidelines-for -avoiding-gluten-unsafe-ingredients-for-gluten-sensitivity/.

Guandalini, Stefano. "A Brief History of Celiac Disease." *Impact: A Publication of the University of Chicago Celiac Disease Center* 7, no. 3 (Summer 2007): 1–2. https://www.cureceliacdisease.org/wp-content/uploads/SU07CeliacCtr.News_.pdf.

Liu, Edwin, Fran Dong, Anna E. Barón, Iman Taki, Jill M. Norris, Brigitte I. Frohnert, Edward J. Hoffenberg, and Marian Rewers. "High Incidence of Celiac Disease in a Long-Term Study of Adolescents with Susceptibility Genotypes." *Gastroenterology* 152, no. 6 (May 2017). doi: 10.1053/j.gastro.2017.02.002.

Offord, Catherine. "The Celiac Surge." *The Scientist* (June 2017). https://www.the -scientist.com/features/the-celiac-surge-31438.

Ratner, Amy. "Nexvax2 Trial Discontinued." *Beyond Celiac*, June 25, 2019. www.beyondceliac.org/research-news/nexvax-2-trial-discontinued/.

Shah, Sveta, and Daniel Leffler. "Celiac Disease: An Underappreciated Issue in Women's Health." *Women's Health* 6, no. 5 (2010): 753–66. doi: 10.2217/WHE.10.57.

The University of Chicago Celiac Disease Center. "Celiac Disease Facts and Figures." Accessed December 10, 2019. https://www.cureceliacdisease.org/wp-content /uploads/341_CDCFactSheets8_FactsFigures.pdf.

INDEX

ACKNOWLEDGMENTS

I would like to thank my husband for being my ultimate sounding board. He always has the best advice when my ideas are off point. I know he supports all my endeavors and encourages me to be a better person. I am so thankful to have him in my life.

I would like to thank my girls for supporting me while I was writing this book. Even though I tried to still be the best mom possible, I know there were times I was extremely busy, and I appreciate not only the support, but also the patience. I love you all so much!

I would like to thank all my gluten-free family members and friends, who are my biggest cheerleaders and tell me all the time how delicious my gluten-free food tastes.

I would like to thank Brenda Kohn, MD, for the remarkable diagnosis of my daughter's celiac disease after so many years when doctors had no answers.

ABOUT THE AUTHOR

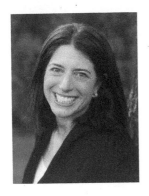 **Jamie Feit, MS, RD,** is a registered dietitian who teaches busy parents how to prepare healthy gluten-free and kosher foods their families will enjoy, without spending hours in the kitchen. With a master's degree in clinical nutrition from New York University, she's been helping her patients meet their nutrition goals for over 20 years.

Jamie has worked with the prestigious Mount Sinai Medical Center, Blythedale Children's Hospital, and Westmed. She now runs her own private practice in New York. She lives with her husband, their four girls, and a large Bernedoodle in Westchester, New York. She observes kosher laws in her home; all nonkosher recipes in this book have substitutions available for ingredients that are not kosher.

You can find more information on Jamie and her practice on her website: www.jamiefeitnutrition.com.